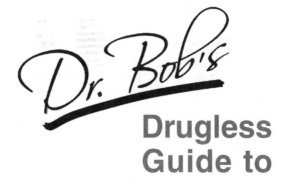

Drugless Guide to

DETOXIFICATION

Books by Dr. Robert DeMaria

Dr. Bob's Drugless Guide to Detoxification

Dr. Bob's Guide to Optimal Health

Available From Destiny Image Publishers

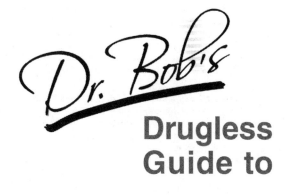

Drugless
Guide to

DETOXIFICATION

Dr. Robert DeMaria

It is not Destiny Image's intention to provide specific medical advice or products, rather this book provides information from Dr. Robert DeMaria for readers' to better understand their health and alternative approaches related to treatment, prevention, screening, and supportive care. Destiny Image urges readers to consult with a qualified healthcare professional for diagnosis and answers to their personal medical questions.

DESTINY IMAGE® PUBLISHERS, INC.
P.O. Box 310, Shippensburg, PA 17257-0310

"Speaking to the Purposes of God for this Generation and for the Generations to Come."

This book and all other Destiny Image, Revival Press, Mercy Place, Fresh Bread, Destiny Image Fiction, and Treasure House books are available at Christian bookstores and distributors worldwide.

For a U.S. bookstore nearest you, **call 1-800-722-6774.**

For more information on foreign distributors, **call 717-532-3040.**

Or reach us on the Internet: **www.destinyimage.com**

ISBN 10: 0-7684-2744-4

ISBN 13: 978-0-7684-2744-8

For Worldwide Distribution, Printed in the U.S.A.

1 2 3 4 5 6 7 8 9 10 11 / 13 12 11 10 09

CONTENTS

In this day and age everyone who has a thought about health asks me, "Dr. Bob, how do I detoxify?" My common response is, "Stop putting toxins in your body." Patients who finally make it to my practice after years of wandering aimlessly looking for answers about how to "clean up their act" are always overjoyed to realize that they can help themselves in the comfort of their own homes.

You will have positive, overall healthy results by adding to your daily routine some simple modifications found in this book. In a relatively short period of time you can achieve restoration of vitality and health. Take it from me—the feeling is terrific!

Dr. Bob's Drugless Guide to Detoxification is designed to give you logical answers to tough questions that you may have wanted to ask but never had the chance. I have created strategies that are simple to follow. My first suggestion is that you read the entire book. Do not make any changes in your lifestyle until you have a good grasp on what your plan will be. Do not arbitrarily or suddenly throw food out of your pantry and risk making your family angry with you.

Take the time to carefully complete the toxicity questionnaire in Chapter 1, which gives you an idea about where you actually are regarding detoxification. Successful results rely on going slowly. Detoxification is not a diet; it is a lifestyle—an enduring change in your life and an extended journey with a happy ending. You *can* regain your optimal health once again.

I would like to caution you, however. You will encounter some individuals along the way who will try to discourage you on this journey. Unfortunately, I have found far too many individuals who want to attain a level of health without making necessary modifications which create optimal cellular function. If you have a circle of friends who are not supportive of your changes, it may be time to look for a healthy circle of influence. Keep in mind that you will become as the group you hang out with. Friends and acquaintances tend to go to the same places to eat after work, drink the same beverages, exercise (or not), and do the same outside activities.

You will want to start exercising a bit more, drinking more water from a pure source, eating organic whole foods, and changing the way you think about what you put in and on your body. Your choices of food and drink will either increase or decrease the energy in your battery, so choose wisely. Do not think that you are above natural principles; everybody's cells function the same way. They are interdependent with each other. Your goal is for your body to function optimally

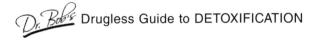

with unprecedented precision without pain, congestion, or lack of energy.

The good news is that over time you will become the glowing lighthouse beacon for many people in and out of your circle; you will become their model and pillar to make it happen for them. So...*go for it!*

Chapter 1

IS YOUR BODY A TOXIC WASTE DUMP?

We live in an increasingly toxic environment. Proliferating nuclear waste, growing landfills, and pollution of our air, land, and water all pose significant external challenges to the health and well-being of people worldwide. Even greater than the threat of *external* toxins, however, are *internal* toxins: poisons and other unhealthy substances we take into our bodies on a daily basis, not only through prescription and non-prescription medications, but also through the food we consume and the beverages we swallow. A large part of the health problems Americans suffer from today are due, at least to some degree, to our habitual consumption of substances that are toxic to the body.

Consider the following. Annually, on average, Americans consume the following:

- 28 pounds per person of French fries. In fact, the French fry is now the number one "vegetable" in America![1]

- 10 billion donuts per year. The ingredients in donuts interfere with fat in the brain and also tax the liver.[2] I fondly call donuts "torpedos of death," they are by far, a distressful source of liver and gall bladder distress.

- 54 gallons of soda pop per person.[3]

- 150-200 pounds of sugar per person. Refined, processed sugar depletes the body of minerals as well as B vitamins and other important enzymes. B vitamins are critical for liver function.[4]

Over a lifetime, we also consume quite a bit of lipstick and lip balm. And don't forget body lotions, hand creams, and sunscreen, as well as prescription and non-prescription medications, all of which introduce foreign chemical substances into the body, which it then must detoxify.

- According to Meg Cohen Ragas and Karen Kozlowski in their book *Read My Lips: A Cultural History of Lipstick*, a reddish purple mercuric plant dye called focus—algin, 0.01 percent iodine, and some bromine mannite—was used for lip rouge by the Egyptians. Little did the ancient Egyptians know that it was potentially poisonous—talk about the kiss of death!

- At least 1.5 million Americans are estimated to be harmed each year from prescription medication errors.[5]

- Over half of Americans are on chronic medications.[6]

- There is the presence of pharmaceuticals in the nation's municipal drinking water supply.

Studies suggest a possible correlation between snack food consumption and incidence of ADHD. The majority of snack foods per captia are consumed in Michigan, Ohio, and Indiana, which, according to a DEA report released years ago, are also the states with the highest levels of use of the psychoactive drug Ritalin.[7]

What causes a contaminated state? As I said before, we have a toxic state because of the water we drink, the food we eat, and the air we inhale. Add to that our general lack of mobility and minimal amount of exercise. A huge problem today for both men and women is an excess of the female hormone estrogen. You can reduce estrogen by focusing on organic food, cleaning up your liver, and making sure you have enough B vitamins. Much of the food we munch on throughout the day is loaded with chemicals that cause us to become addicted to those food items. This is particularly true with snack and junk food. Addiction to these kinds of foods feeds the spiraling epidemic of obesity in this country.

One simple solution is to focus on organic food. Once exotic in both reputation and price, organic food today is available at very affordable prices from major marketers such as Wal-Mart. Because it is designed to be free of chemicals, additives, preservatives, or anything else artificial, organic food is a sensible and basic step in detoxifying the body.

Detoxification = Purification

A synonym, in the context of this book, for detoxification is *purification*. Many practitioners of modern medicine do not really understand the importance of purification. It is not commonly part of their medical training and therefore is not a major concern for them. Although there are many signs that the picture is starting to change, the primary focus of modern medicine is on *treatment* rather than *prevention*. The sobering truth is that many of the treatment protocols others recommend actually create a toxic environment. For example, one alarming statistic has estimated that over three years, 600,000 people die from medical errors.[8]

In its report, "To Err Is Human: Building a Safer Health System," the Institute of

Medicine (IOM) estimates that 44,000 to 98,000 Americans die each year not from medical conditions, but from preventable medical errors.

The IOM estimates that fully half of adverse reactions to medicines are the result of medical errors. Other adverse reactions—those that are unexpected and not preventable—are not considered errors. (See "When Is a Medical Product Too Risky?" in the September–October 1999 issue of *FDA Consumer*.)

From my experience many senior citizens who come into the office take aspirin as a blood thinner. It is used to treat and help prevent heart attacks, but aspirin is toxic to the liver. Acetaminophen (Tylenol), on the other hand, is toxic for the kidneys. Thick blood is a problem for many people today, and one of the primary causes of thick blood is the partially hydrogenated oils, or *trans fat*, found in so many snack foods, and is part of the long-term toxic challenge for all ages. From my experience and understanding physiology, aspirin does not in actuality get to the cause of the problem of thick blood. We often have thick blood because we have too much inflammation inside our bodies. Patients who are taking aspirin appear to have chronic black and blue skin bruising on their arms and hands because the aspirin is disrupting normal cell physiology to an extreme.

Medical errors involving seniors is quite substantial. The additional cost to taxpayers to treat Medicare patients who were victims of medical errors, including those who lived and died, is about $2.9 billion a year.[9]

Bile, which is released by the gallbladder, is a vital component that helps maintain blood coagability or "thinness." The ancient Greeks were among the first to explore the nature and function of bodily fluids, including bile and blood. In fact, the Greeks identified four critical bodily fluids, which they called *humors*: yellow bile, black bile, blood, and phlegm. They were interested in how fluids moved in the body, as well as the role those fluids played in regulating one's health. It was their belief that a healthy

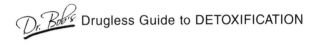

person was one in whom the four humors were in proper balance. Consequently, Hippocrates and other ancient healers sought ways to bring about that balance in their patients. For this purpose they incorporated a variety of methods, including fasting, massage, acupuncture, saunas, and baths. While the ancient Greeks may have gotten a lot of things incorrect about human anatomy and physiology, one thing they got right was the importance of balance. A toxic body is a body out of balance.

Detoxification, or purification, is the process of bringing a toxic body back into balance by eliminating the poisons that have overloaded bodily organs and upset the body's equilibrium.

Common Signs of Toxicity

Toxicity in the body reveals itself in many different ways. The key is discovering what to look for. Skin eruptions of most types including severe acne is one example. Acne is a common challenge among children going through hormonal changes of puberty, but it can be a marker of liver function. Chronic acne and skin challenges are an over-looked body signal that the liver is not functioning optimally, which often is due to dysfunction with resulting toxicity in the colon.

A 10-year-old girl with severe acne came into my office as a new patient. Before coming to us she had been to three endocrinologists and several other healthcare providers—each labeling her condition differently—and had found no relief. I recommended that she start drinking a minimum of one quart of water a day.

Why water? The key organ in the body that should be free of toxins is the colon. This young girl was having a bowel movement only once every two to three days. Healthy children her age should be so regular as to have a bowel movement within an hour or two after every meal. In fact, healthy adults should normally have a minimum of three bowel movements a day. Moving bowels only once every two or three days is a body signal of poor detoxification function.

Water helps flush out toxins, cleanse the colon, and regulate bowel elimination. A sluggish colon affects the liver. The liver is one of the keys to the body's ability to detoxify itself. A lethargic colon can precipitate the factors for the liver to become congested and cease to function as efficiently as it should. A stagnant or impaired liver soon compromises the kidneys, which are also critical for toxin and waste elimination.

People with high blood pressure usually are instructed not to eat salt. But salt is often not the root of the problem. Frequently high blood pressure occurs because the liver is toxic and the kidneys are trying to make up the difference. The resulting backup of toxins often manifests on the skin, as with acne. Another telltale sign of a toxicity problem which is appearing more and more often on younger people is brown spots on the skin. Popularly called "age or liver spots," these brown marks are not limited to elderly people but are characteristic of people with liver problems. One common cause is an insufficient level of vitamin E in the liver. Vitamin E is a nutrient needed for many functions including the pituitary gland; too little of it prevents the liver from eliminating toxins sufficiently, resulting in brown spots. Brown spots on the skin may be a sign that the liver is not functioning at peak performance.

Similarly, acne often results from a hormonal imbalance, which suggests that the liver is not functioning properly. In addition to drinking plenty of water, another good protocol is to eat an apple a day, preferably with the peel that has been washed. Fuji or Gala apples are preferred. For breakfast, especially for children, a warm stewed apple with some cinnamon on it tastes great, is filling, and will start their digestion working properly for the day.

Other body signals of toxicity include psoriasis and eczema, both of which are markers that the skin is being used as a dumping ground, and are also symptoms of liver function. Profuse sweating, particularly of the feet, while often symptomatic of an adrenal gland problem (a pair of glands located on top of the kidneys which control mineral balance in the body), can also be caused by a stagnant liver and kidney.

Chronic bad breath is also a signal of toxicity. Bad breath relief is a humongous industry in America. Most "remedies" target the symptom rather than the source. Persistent, nasty, sewer-smelling breath hardly ever originates in the mouth. Usually it results from the decomposition of food that is improperly or insufficiently digested. It is like having a compost pile in your stomach, and the odor rises up through the esophagus and into the mouth. Incomplete and inefficient digestion commonly results from not enough digestive enzymes and acid with inadequate acid and then combined with impaired liver and/or a sluggish colon. These conditions may result from the presence of toxins in the body from poor digestion and in these organs, which create chemical imbalances that hinder proper function including digestion.

Taking an antacid versus getting to the cause of the problem is not helpful. I encourage my patients to avoid drinking fluids with their meals, or keep liquids to a minimum. Do not drink cold water, and for digestive purposes never eat cold leftovers—they are a poor source of energy and will stagnate digestion.

Where do you stand on the toxicity scale? How toxic is your body? An honest self-assessment is important to determining a course of action. For this reason, take time to complete the following Toxicity Questionnaire. Be honest with yourself. It's important to know where you are before you can determine where you need to go to become a healthier you.

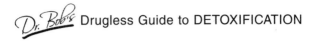

Toxicity Questionnaire[10]

Section I: Symptoms

Rate each of the following based upon your health profile for the past 90 days.

Circle the corresponding number.

0   Rarely or never experience the symptom

1   Occasionally experience the symptom; effect is not severe

2   Occasionally experience the symptom; effect is severe

3   Frequently experience the symptom; effect is not severe

4   Frequently experience the symptom; effect is severe

1. DIGESTIVE

a.	Nausea and/or vomiting		(0)	1	2	3	4
b.	Diarrhea		0	(1)	2	3	4
c.	Constipation		(0)	1	2	3	4
d.	Bloated feeling		(0)	1	2	3	4
e.	Belching and/or passing gas		0	(1)	2	3	4
f.	Heartburn		(0)	1	2	3	4

Total: _2_

2. EARS

a.	Itchy ears		(0)	1	2	3	4
b.	Earaches, ear infections		(0)	1	2	3	4
c.	Drainage from ear		(0)	1	2	3	4
d.	Ringing in ears, hearing loss		0	(1)	2	3	4

Total: _1_

3. EMOTIONS

a. Mood swings	0 ①2 3 4
b. Anxiety, fear, nervousness	0 1 2 ③4
c. Anger, irritability	0 ①2 3 4
d. Depression	⓪1 2 3 4
e. Sense of despair	⓪1 2 3 4
f. Apathy/lethargy	⓪1 2 3 4

Total: _____5_____

4. ENERGY/ACTIVITY

a. Fatigue/sluggishness	0 ①2 3 4
b. Hyperactivity	0 1 ②3 4
c. Restlessness	0①2 3 4
d. Insomnia	⓪1 2 3 4
e. Startled awake at night	0①2 3 4

Total: _____5_____

5. EYES

a.	Watery, itchy eyes	(0) 1 2 3 4
b.	Swollen, reddened, or sticky eyelids	(0) 1 2 3 4
c.	Dark circles under eyes	(0) 1 2 3 4
d.	Blurred/tunnel vision	0 (1) 2 3 4

Total: _____

6. HEAD

a.	Headaches	0 (1) 2 3 4
b.	Faintness	(0) 1 2 3 4
c.	Dizziness	(0) 1 2 3 4
d.	Pressure	0 (1) 2 3 4

Total: ___2___

7. LUNGS

a.	Chest congestion	0	1	2	3	4
b.	Asthma, Bronchitis	0	1	2	3	4
c.	Shortness of breath	0	1	2	3	4
d.	Difficulty breathing	0	1	2	3	4

Total: _____

8. MIND

a.	Poor memory	0	①(1)	2	3	4
b.	Confusion	0	1	2	3	4
c.	Poor concentration	0	1	2	3	4
d.	Poor coordination	0	1	2	3	4
e.	Difficulty making decisions	0	1	2	3	4
f.	Stuttering, stammering	0	1	2	3	4
g.	Slurred speech	0	1	2	3	4
h.	Learning disabilities	0	1	2	3	4

Total: _____

9. MOUTH/THROAT

a.	Chronic coughing		0 1 2 3 4
b.	Gagging, frequent need to clear throat		0 1 2 3 4
c.	Swollen or discolored tongue, gums, lips		0 1 2 3 4
d.	Canker sores		0 1 2 3 4
		Total:	◯

10. NOSE

a.	Stuffy nose		0 ①2 3 4
b.	Sinus problems		0 1 2 3 4
c.	Hay fever		0 1 2 3 4
d.	Sneezing attacks		0 1 2 3 4
e.	Excessive mucous		0 ①2 3 4
		Total:	2

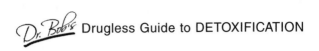

11. SKIN

a.	Acne	0 1 2 3 ④
b.	Hives, rashes, dry skin	0 1 2 3 4
c.	Hair loss	0 1 2 3 4
d.	Flushing	0 1 2 3 4
e.	Excessive sweating	0 1 2 3 4

Total: 4

12. HEART

a.	Skipped heartbeats	0 ① 2 3 4
b.	Rapid heartbeats	0 1 2 3 4
c.	Chest pain	0 1 2 3 4

Total: 1

13. JOINTS / MUSCLES

a.	Pain or aches in joints	0	1	2	3	4
b.	Rheumatoid arthritis	0	1	2	3	4
c.	Osteoarthritis	0	1	2	3	4
d.	Stiffness, limited movement	0	1	2	3	4
e.	Pain, aches in muscles	0	1	2	3	4
f.	Recurrent back aches	0	1	2	3	4
g.	Feeling of weakness or tiredness	0	1	2	3	4

Total: ___

14. WEIGHT

a.	Binge eating/drinking	0	(1)	2	3	4
b.	Craving certain foods	0	1	2	3	4
c.	Excessive weight	0	1	2	3	4
d.	Compulsive eating	0	(1)	2	3	4
e.	Water retention	0	1	2	3	4
f.	Underweight	0	1	2	3	4

Total: ___

15. OTHER

a.	Frequent illness	0 1 2 3 4
b.	Frequent or urgent urination	0 1 2 3 4
c.	Leaky bladder	0 1 2 3 4
d.	Genital itch, discharge	0 1 2 3 4

Total: _0_

Section I Total: _26_

Section II: Risk of Exposure

Rate each of the following situations based upon your environmental profile for the past 120 days.

16. Circle the corresponding number for questions 16a–16f.

0   Never

1   Rarely

2   Monthly

3   Weekly

4   Daily

a.   How often are strong chemicals used in your home? (disinfectants, bleaches, oven & drain cleaners, furniture polish, floor wax, window cleaners, etc.)

0 ① 2 3 4

b.   How often are pesticides used in your home?

⓪ 1 2 3 4

c.   How often do you have your home treated for insects?

⓪ 1 2 3 4

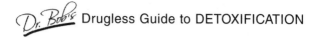

d. How often are you exposed to dust, over-stuffed furniture, tobacco smoke, mothballs, incense, or varnish in your home or office?

(0) 1 2 3 4

e. How often are you exposed to nail polish, perfume, hair spray, and other cosmetics?

0 (1) 2 3 4

f. How often are you exposed to diesel fumes, exhaust fumes, or gasoline fumes?

(0) 1 2 3 4

Total: 2

17. Circle the corresponding number for questions 17a–17b below.

0   No

1   Mild Change

2   Moderate Change

3   Drastic Change

a. Have you noticed any negative change in your health since you moved into your home or apartment?

0 1 ② 3

b. Have you noticed any negative change in your health since you started your new job?

⓪ 1 2 3

Total:	
Section II Total:	
Total from Section I & II:	

How did you do? If you had a score lower than 30, you are doing well. If your score was higher than 30, you will want to think about some type of detoxification program. Also, if you score more than six on three or more groups, you will want to evaluate your health habits.

If you discovered that you have some toxicity issues, don't despair. Almost everyone does. The good news is that you can do something about it. As I said before, many of the treatment protocols of modern medicine can add to the problem rather than alleviate it, because the focus is on treatment of the symptoms rather than detoxifying the body. Informed healthcare providers, like myself and others, incorporate less dangerous items, such as selected nutrients, including whole foods, supplements, and herbs.

Synthetic high-potency vitamins can cause distress. Many people come into my office with bags and boxes of supplements that they take regularly, but they still feel lousy. If you have been taking supplements, you are better off putting them away, eating whole foods, and allowing your body the opportunity to heal itself.

The following chapters provide tested, proven, commonsense, *natural* ways to detoxify your body and restore proper balance *without* drugs. Your body wants to heal itself, and our Creator built into it the ability to do just that. The key to success is your willingness to change your way of thinking as well as a willingness to make the necessary changes in your lifestyle and habits to promote *natural* wellness.

Are you ready? Then let's get down to business.

Just Tell Me What to Do!

• Drink water from a pure source. I encourage my patients to drink reverse osmosis water. Eat raw, steamed, and sautéed organic veggies for minerals and to keep your pH at the right level.

- Avoid all soft drinks and fruit drinks with artificial sweeteners, including aspartame (NutraSweet), sucralose (Splenda), HFCS or high fructose corn syrup. Also avoid additives that have been developed that create sweetness.

- Eat Dr. Bob's ABCs every day. Eat one half of a red apple; one-third cup of organic raw grated, baked, pressure-cooked, or steamed beets; and five baby organic or one medium carrot daily. These items promote optimal liver function.

- Read labels; avoid foods that have colors added to them. It is best to eat organic foods.

- Use Celtic Sea Salt for flavoring. It has not been tampered like other commercial products.

- Take one tablespoon of flax oil a day per 100 pounds of body weight. Flax oil is a great pain reliever. You can also grind flax seeds and add them to your salads, squashes, and brown rice.

- Get to bed by 10 P.M. Sleep promotes healing and restoration.

- Take 20 every day. Twenty minutes of some type of activity gets the lymph and blood flowing in your body. Motion is life and will help move the "humors" our predecessors discussed.

Endnotes

1. Consumption of French fries, http://findarticles.com/p/articles/mi_m0DQA/is_2002_Feb_28/ai_83663496.

2. Sally Levitt Steinberg, *The Donut Book* (North Adams, MA, 2004).

3. CSPI Center of Science in Public Interest. Newsroom Report July 13, 2005.

4. Vikki Conwell, "The American Dietetic Association," Cox News Service, *The Plain Dealer*, May 30, 2007.

5. Laruan Neerguard, "Prescription name game can be deadly," *Chronicle Telegram,* September 2, 2008.

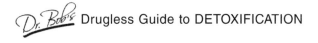

6. Linda Johnson, *The Morning Journal*, May 14, 2008.

7. DEA and Ritalin: *The Cleveland Plain Dealer,* Sunday, May 6, 2001, "Ritalin Prescriptions Vary Widely." "Fatal Medical Errors Said to Be More Widespread," by Paul Davies. *The Wall Street Journal* July 27, 2004. Based on a study by Health Grades Inc. a health care consulting firm in Colorado that rates hospitals.

8. Paul Davies, *Wall Street Journal*.

9. *U.S. Preventive Services Task Force Urges Clinicians and Patients to Discuss Aspirin Therapy.* Press Release, January 14, 2002. Agency for Healthcare Research and Quality, Rockville, MD; http://www.ahrq.gov/news/press/pr2002/aspirpr.htm.

10. Adapted with permission from the author, Dr. Gina L. Nick, from *Clinical Purification™: A Complete Treatment and Reference Manual.*

11. Martha Mendoza, "Drugs in water report leads to calls for action." *The Elyria Chronicle Telegram*, AP. March 17, 2008.

12. Paul Davies, "Fatal Medical Errors said to be more widespread." *Wall Street Journal*, July 27, 2004.

Chapter 2

YOU ARE
WHAT YOU EAT

Were you surprised by the results of the Toxicity Questionnaire in the previous chapter? Perhaps you discovered that your body scored low on the toxicity scale. If so, I applaud you and encourage you to continue making good choices regarding diet, exercise, and other factors that keep your toxic levels low. At the same time, I encourage you to keep reading, because you may very well discover additional steps you can take and changes you can make that will reduce your toxicity even more. Our goal should always be to reduce the toxicity in our bodies to the lowest possible level—and keep it there. (See

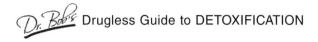

Appendix D, Detoxification Food Selection and Consumption.)

If you are historically like a number of people who present to my office however, the questionnaire revealed that your body is toxic enough to warrant a cleansing protocol. You may be asking, "Why am I toxic? How did I get this way, and how can I change it?"

To begin with, it is important to understand where toxicity comes from. Once you know *how* you became toxic, it will be easier for you to understand how to detoxify as well as how to prevent it from happening again. So let's start by talking about the most common sources of toxins in the body.

Food Additives

Food additives have become so thoroughly ingrained into the American food industry that they seem almost impossible to avoid. In today's society, certified organically grown food is just about the only additive-free source of nutrition. But until very recent years organic food has been too expensive for many Americans to buy extensively on a regular basis.

What's wrong with food additives? Why are they such a concern? Food additives are chemical substances added to food to preserve it from spoilage, improve appearance, enhance flavor, and generally make the food more appealing overall. The problem with additives is that often they are approved for use before adequate testing has demonstrated that they possess no negative side effects or pose any long-term health risks. In some cases, additives long accepted as harmless and "nontoxic" have proven to be otherwise as more information has come to light. Common artificial food coloring is one prime example.

According to the nonprofit Center for Science in the Public Interest, (CSPI)Yellow 5, Red 40, and six other widely used artificial colorings have been linked to hyperactivity and behavior problems in children and should be prohibited from use in foods. To this end,

CSPI formally petitioned the Food and Drug Administration to ban the dyes, several of which are already being phased out in the United Kingdom. The other six dyes in question are Blue 1, Blue 2, Green 3, Orange B, Red 3, and Yellow 6.

"The continued use of these unnecessary artificial dyes is the secret shame of the food industry and the regulators who watch over it," said CSPI executive director Michael F. Jacobson. "The purpose of these chemicals is often to mask the absence of real food, to increase the appeal of a low-nutrition product to children, or both. Who can tell the parents of kids with behavioral problems that this is truly worth the risk?"[1]

Americans' exposure to artificial food dyes has risen sharply over the years. According to the FDA, the amount of food dye certified for use in 1955 was 12 milligrams per capita per day. In 2007, 59 mg per capita per day, or nearly five times as much, was certified for use. Dyes are used in countless foods and are sometimes used to simulate the color of fruits or vegetables. For example, a popular guacamole dip gets its greenish color not from avocados (there are almost none) but from Yellow 5, Yellow 6, and Blue 1. The blue bits in some blueberry waffles are not real blueberries but coloration due to Red 40 and Blue 2.

Americans' exposure to artificial food dyes has risen sharply over the years.

The following information is taken from the Center for Science in the Public Interest, *Nutrition Action*, April 2008. Artificial dyes are particularly prevalent in the sugary cereals, candies, sodas, and snack foods pitched to kids. For instance, General Mills' Fruit Roll-ups and Fruit-by-the-Foot flavored snacks get their fruity colors from Yellow 5, Yellow 6, Red 40, and Blue 1. Their Fruity Cheerios, Lucky Charms, and Trix also contain several of the problematic dyes, as do Kellogg's Froot Loops and Apple Jacks and Post's Fruity Pebbles.

More than a dozen American varieties of Kraft's Oscar Meyer Lunchables kids' meals contain artificial food dyes, *but not so the British versions*. Starburst Chews, Skittles, and M&M candies—all Mars products—contain the full spectrum of artificial colors in the U.S., but not in the U.K., where the company uses natural colorings. Even foods that aren't particularly brightly colored can contain dyes, including several varieties of macaroni and cheese and mashed potatoes.

For instance, Betty Crocker's Au Gratin "100% Real" Potatoes are partly not real, colored as they are with Yellow 5 and Yellow 6, both of which are derived from coal tar. Remarkably, in Britain, the color in McDonald's strawberry sauce for sundaes actually comes from strawberries; in the U.S. the color comes from Red 40.

"The science shows that kids' behavior improves when these artificial colorings are removed from their diets and worsens when they're added to the their diets," said Dr. David Schab, a psychiatrist at Columbia

University Medical Center, who conducted a 2004 meta-analysis with his colleague Dr. Nhi-Ha T. Trinh. "While not all children seem to be sensitive to these chemicals," he continued, "it's hard to justify their continued use in foods—especially those foods heavily marketed to young children."

Many companies change formulas when under pressure from the government and consumers.

Secretive Chemicals

As if this were not bad enough, today it is increasingly likely that "secretive" chemicals are being hidden in food under the designation of "artificial flavors." A relatively young company, Senomyx, may be responsible for the sodium and sugar levels falling in many of our favorite grocery store items. How?

Senomyx has contracted with Kraft, Nestle, Coca Cola, and Campbell Soup to put a chemical in foods that masks bitter flavors by turning off bitter flavor receptors on the tongue and enhancing salty and sweet flavors. This allows companies to tout claims such as "less sugar" or "lower sodium" by reducing the actual sugar and/or salt in their foods by approximately half while retaining the same level of sweetness or saltiness when they touch the tongue. The chemical additives fool the brain into thinking that the sweetness is the same.

Mark Zoller, Senomyx's chief scientist, says that his company has used the human genome sequence to identify hundreds of taste receptors. Senomyx's chemical compounds enhance those receptors to heighten the taste of salt or sugar. Under this premise, they claim that their newly added chemicals are completely safe because they will be used in tiny quantities of less than one part per million whereas artificial sweeteners are used in 200–500 parts per million. This fact alone allows them to forgo the rigorous FDA approval process normally required before introducing new food additives into the marketplace. Attaining the status of GRAS (generally recognized as safe) from the Flavor and

Extract Manufacturers Association i
most advanced product, which replace   ᴜɢ,
took the company less than 18 months. Their
evidence? Results of a three-month safety
study conducted on rats.

After pouring a total of 30 million dollars
into research and development, the companies that have invested in *Senomyx's*
products have been secretive, to say the
least, about their involvement with the
company. Some, like Kraft, have declined
to divulge any specifics regarding their
relationship with *Senomyx* but instead
stated that Kraft was committed "to reducing the sugar and salt levels in many products." Nestle and Coca Cola declined to
comment. I think silence says it all.[2]

In addition to the artificial colorings mentioned above, other common food additives
that are best avoided include:

- Sodium Nitrate

- BHA and BHT

- Propyl Gallate

- Sosodium Glutamate

- Aspartame

- Acesulfame – K

- Olestra

- Potassium Bromate

- White sugar

- Sodium Chloride

There is one food additive that is so ubiquitous in our culture and so detrimental to our overall health that we need to give it some special attention. I'm talking about partially hydrogenated oils, also known as *trans fat*.

The Problem of Trans Fat

Millions of Americans today are misinformed regarding the merits and dangers of fat in their diet and are suffering the consequences. Manmade fat modification, industrial fat alteration, and media fat misinformation together have had an enormous negative impact on our current level of health.

Because of a general misunderstanding of fat and the role it plays in our bodies, people are dying, disabled, chemically dependent, surgically altered, and living daily in pain. Many physical ailments, including hormonal imbalances, can be attributed to poor fat function. Our bodies *need* fat for optimal health and wellness.

As with anything else, the key to understanding fat is knowledge. It is important, therefore, to learn the names of different kinds of fats and their activities in order to make logical and wise decisions about what to eat. Like them or not, fats are crucial to our bodies for helping to build cells, tissues, organs, and hormones. Cell membranes are made of fat. In fact, it is accurate to say that the quality of our cells is dependent on the fat we eat—or don't eat!

Saturated fats are solid at room temperature. They can be derived from both plant and animal sources, although most come from animal sources. For many years saturated fat has been branded as "bad" fat for its role as a major factor in causing high cholesterol and heart disease. Less well-known is the fact that saturated animal fat also contains "healthy" monounsaturated fats. By itself, saturated fat is not bad, but only part of a bigger picture in heart and other health problems.

Monounsaturated fats are liquid at room temperatures and thicken in the refrigerator. One example is olive oil. It can be heated to moderate temperatures and is great for sautéing food. It also tastes great in place of butter on a huge variety of foods. Oleic acid is another monounsaturated fat. Found in olive, almond, pistachio, pecan, avocado, hazelnut, cashew and macadamia oils, as well as in the membranes of plant and animal cell structures, oleic acid helps keep arteries supple.

Polyunsaturated fats are liquid. They do not get hard at room temperature and remain liquid in cool environments.

Fats and oils found in nature, in their raw, uncooked state, are neither bad nor good. Heat modifies fat molecules in mono and polyunsaturated fats. Imbalanced fat eating (with either a heavy focus on saturated and heated vegetable oils) is what creates a scenario for unhealthy bodies. The "low fat" that has been such a craze over the last decade or two is actually trans fat, which creates inflammation in the body, especially when compounded (as it almost always is) with high levels of sugar to enhance flavor. The low-fat, high-carbohydrate diet was created to lower cholesterol, under the premise that there was no cholesterol in the plant-sourced oils. Trans fat is the principal culprit, the primary fire that is fueling the rise of health-related crises such as obesity, diabetes, heart disease, and cancer.

Consequently, trans fat, or partially hydrogenated oils, has become one of the leading health challenges facing our society today. These manmade oils have permeated nearly every aspect of our modern food chain. They have also created havoc in the detoxifying organs (liver, colon, kidneys). Because of all the misinformation and alarmist literature related to fat, Americans have created a "fat phobia" epidemic. Confusion is rampant. To cut through the fog, remember first that *fat or*

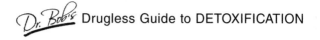

oil is not the enemy! The problem lies in the *kinds* of fats or oils we choose. We need to make wise selections. Food manufacturers and restaurants are scurrying to find an alternative for the oils they fry and cook with, while maintaining an appealing taste and keeping their profit margins up. Why? Because better educated consumers are demanding healthier ingredients. Knowledge is a powerful thing.

Trans fat is the villain of the day.

Trans fat is the villain of the day. It all started in Europe in 1873, when in an effort to find a new source for candle wax, the first "batch" of partially hydrogenated oil was developed. The American public had its first taste of mass-produced "oleomargarine" during World War II. Despite popular perception and marketing claims to the contrary, margarine is *not* a viable replacement for butter.

Partially hydrogenated oil (trans fat) is made by heating vegetable oil at very high temperatures. Part of the process involves pumping hydrogen into the container in the presence of a metal catalyst, stopping right before *full* loading of the hydrogen has occurred; hence the name "partially hydrogenated." The exact final result of the process is not completely known. Trans fat is one of the by-products of this process. Full hydrogenation would result in a solid substance. Partially hydrogenated fat is not solid at room temperatures.

The trans fat dilemma arose in part out of the desire to reduce the incidence of heart disease, to which high cholesterol was considered the major contributing factor. Vegetable oil does not have cholesterol in it. Animal products do. Seventy percent of the current oil used in the United States is soy based. Soy oil is commonly extracted from the bean using hexane. I do not recommend soy oil or products. During the fat phobia years, people were told to avoid products and processes made with animal tissue (i.e., lard, beef tallow, cheese, heavy dairy cream, and eggs). Conventional medicine took the view that if the public would stop eating those foods, the

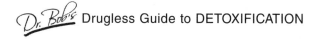

high instance of heart attacks would decrease. What most people do not realize, however, is that the human body makes up to 75 percent of its cholesterol on a "make as you need, supply and demand basis." Cholesterol is essential for our survival as a species; it is a precursor for sex hormones. Vegetable-based fat or oils do not have cholesterol.

LDL and HDL

Originally, trans fat was regarded as not being true "fat" because it does not have cholesterol. The plan was simple: low fat meant no cholesterol, which meant reduced danger of heart attack and other heart disease. The low fat/no fat diet fad began. All you have to do is look around to see that this plan has not worked successfully. People are heavier now than ever, and heart disease and heart attacks are the leading cause of death in the Western world. America has been on the low fat "kick" for nearly 40 years, and people are still dying of heart disease!

Keep in mind that the low fat diet is loaded with trans fat with sugar added to enhance flavor and taste. This deadly combination did not help lower cholesterol like everyone thought it would. Instead, it actually *raised* the level of LDL (perceived as the bad) cholesterol while lowering the level of HDL (considered the good) cholesterol.

Cholesterol is not water soluble and cannot easily be transported in blood without assistance. Cholesterol is not really bad or good, but necessary. It acts like a fire fighter. When there is a fire or inflammation in the body, cholesterol is called upon to be a building block to make cortisone which assists in dampening the fire. Cortisone stops inflammation. When a person has elevated LDL, the conventional mindset thinks, *Oh! I'm in trouble now.* But the truth is, your body is doing its job creating more cholesterol, which becomes your body's natural firefighter—cortisone—putting out the fire caused commonly by trans fat and sugar. *LDL cholesterol is the fire truck taking cholesterol to the fire, and in reality is doing its job.*

Taking cholesterol-lowering medication with its bad effects will result in the stopping of the natural function of physiology in the body. The real problem of heart disease is continuing in our culture because the public has been misinformed with data about what is causing the inflammation. It is not just red meat and eggs (eggs and red meat are by far the least of your major concern). Stop eating the fake fats, sugar and food additives that alter proper fat metabolism.

Natural vegetable oil unaltered by man will not normally raise cholesterol unless you tend to overeat Omega 6 fats; safflower and sunflower oils are examples.

Omega 6 fats relieve pain while assisting proper blood flow; when they are the primary fat in your diet, which is common, you may have an overflow phenomenon resulting in pain and inflammation. The public currently consumes more Omega 6 versus Omega 3 fats. The ratio generally should be about 1 to 1. Read _Dr. Bob's Trans Fat Survival Guide; Why No_

Fat, Low Fat, Trans Fats are Killing You for more information.

What happens with trans fat or partially hydrogenated oil is the chemical bonds in the fat molecules are altered with heat and the hydrogen and chemical catalyst used in the conversion. The fat molecule from the once-healthy oil creates a physiology predicament at the cellular level. The body then responds with a defense mechanism that raises cholesterol to protect itself.

Fake food generally causes an inflammatory response at the microscopic cell level. Trans fat raises cholesterol because it is one of the primary causes of inflammation. Remember, the body produces cholesterol to protect itself from inflammation. The medical community is doing everything it can to artificially lower their patients' cholesterol levels, which unfortunately includes prescribing unnatural remedies. That is why we have "side effects" with cholesterol-lowering medication. The body can get confused when cholesterol is lowered artificially. Trans fat interferes with

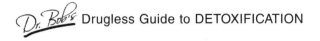

the inflammation-lowering efforts of choles-terol. (See Appendix D, Detoxification Food Selection and Consumption.)

The main problem with trans fat: it attempts to fool mother nature. We live and die at the cellular level. The cells in our body become perplexed when trans fat is hanging around in abundance. In addition to raising LDL (which now you can see why it is per-ceived as bad) cholesterol levels, trans fat cre-ates many other complications. Here are only a few:

- Inflammation response.

- Small holes in the cell membrane.

- Correlates to low birth rate.

- Precipitates childhood asthma.

- Inhibits essential fatty acid metabolism.

- Alters enzyme reactions in the body.

- Decreases the red blood cells' response to insulin.

Small amounts of trans fat are found in nature. Generally the body uses those molecules for energy. When a large quantity of trans fat is present, however, the body starts incorporating it into cellular membranes. This is not good. How does this "fake fat" affect your body? Whenever we eat a meal, our body takes that food and breaks it down. Various nutrients are needed to complete the sequence: B complex, B6, calcium, magnesium, zinc, various enzymes. All these ingredients and others are necessary for the body to do its job.

If one of the components is missing or in short supply, the body suffers. A good example is Vitamin B6, which is commonly low in most people who diet on the run, either by choice or by eating anti-vitamins like sugar. Lack of B6 can, among other things, lead to carpal tunnel or wrist pain symptoms. Without B6, the body does not create enough of a fat tissue hormone called a prostaglandin. The prostaglandin in this case is created to take away inflammation. All of this is a result of poor fat metabolism, which means you can have pain.

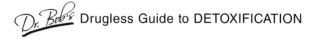

In addition, trans fat interferes with the metabolic pathways that have to do with brain and heart health. Trans fat sabotages the process. Trans fat has a half-life of 51 days. This means that if you eat a food with trans fat or partially hydrogenated fat today, its negative effect will linger in you, with 25 percent of its negative potency, for 102 days. Can you see now how insidiously trans fat can affect your health, particularly if you consume it on a regular basis?

Trans fat is the leading cause of health problems today because it has mysteriously gone undetected for nearly 40 years and has permeated nearly every fabric of our food chain. In January 2006, the federal government required all commercial foods to display on the package the amount of trans fat content. Unfortunately, there is a loophole. A product containing one-half gram or less of trans fat per serving can be legally advertised as containing "0 Grams Trans Fat." When you see "0" on the label, you should turn the package over and read the Nutrition Facts. If you see partially hydrogenated oils, put the package back on the shelf. Trans fats are everywhere: in vitamins, candy, bread, cereal, novelty items—you name it.

We must become label savvy. This is why we are seeing more and more cities voting to remove trans fat from restaurants. A study released in the late 1990s concluded that consuming more than one gram of trans fat a day increases the risk of cardiovascular disease by 20 percent.[3] A new study ties high consumption of trans fat, found mainly in partially hydrogenated vegetable oils and widely used by the food industry, to an increased risk of coronary heart disease (CHD).

The study by the Harvard School of Public Health (HSPH) provides the strongest association to date between trans fat and heart disease. It found that women in the U.S. with the highest levels of trans fat in their blood had three times the risk of CHD as those with the lowest levels.

The study was published online on March 26, 2007, and appeared in the April 10, 2007,

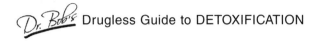

print issue of *Circulation: Journal of the American Heart Association.*

"The strength of this study is that the amount of trans fatty acid levels was measured in blood samples from the study population," said senior author Frank Hu, associate professor of nutrition and epidemiology at HSPH. "Because humans cannot synthesize trans fatty acids, the amount of trans fat in red blood cells is an excellent biomarker of trans fat intake."

Clinical trials have shown that trans fatty acids increase LDL cholesterol and lower HDL cholesterol, making them the only class of fatty acids, which includes saturated fat, to have this dual effect. HDL (high-density lipoprotein) is considered a "good" cholesterol; LDL (low-density lipoprotein) perceived as the "bad" cholesterol.

The researchers, led by Hu and lead author Qi Sun, a graduate research assistant at HSPH, set out to test the assumption that higher trans fatty acid levels in erythrocytes—red blood cells—were associated with a higher risk of heart disease among U.S. women.

Blood samples collected in 1989 and 1990 from 32,826 participants in the Brigham and Women's Hospital-based Nurses' Health Study were examined. During six years of follow-up, 166 cases of CHD were diagnosed and matched with 327 controls for age, smoking status, fasting status and date of blood drawing.

After adjusting for age, smoking status, and other dietary and lifestyle cardiovascular risk factors, the researchers found that a higher level of trans fatty acids in red blood cells was associated with an elevated risk of CHD.

The risk among women in the top quartile of trans fat levels was triple that of the lowest quartile. "Positive associations have been shown in earlier studies based on dietary data provided by the participants, but the use of biomarkers of trans fatty acids is believed to be more reliable than self-reports. This is probably the reason why we see an even stronger

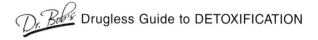

association between blood levels of trans fat and risk of CHD in this study," said Sun.

"These data provide further justifications for current efforts to remove trans fat from foods and restaurant meals," said Hu. "Trans fat intake in the U.S. is still high. Reducing trans fat intake should remain an important public health priority."

The study was supported by the National Institutes of Health.

Trans fat is one of the biggest sources of body toxicity today, which is why any effective detoxification protocol must take into account its presence and negative effects.

Here are a few simple tips for reducing or eliminating trans fat in your body:

- Learn to read ingredient labels.

- Avoid packaged convenience foods: read the label.

- Eat cereals infrequently: read the label.

- Avoid commercial-grade peanut butter with partially hydrogenated or trans fat.

- Avoid or minimize processed food, particularly snack foods, snack cakes, and the like.

Another significant, although lesser known, source of toxicity in the body comes not from additives in the food we eat, but from the containers they are packaged in.

Hard Questions about Hard Plastic

Bisphenol A (BPA) is a hormone disruptor that can be found in almost everybody. Animal studies have linked it to breast and prostate cancer as well as infertility.[4] It affects the body negatively by increasing estrogen to unhealthy levels.

Estrogen overload is a major health challenge today that affects both males and females of all ages. Synthetic estrogens, xenohormones, create imbalances in the body. They are commonly found in polycarbonate, one of the plastics that carry the No.

7 recycling symbol. Polycarbonate is clear, tough, and lightweight, making it ideal for bulletproof glass, water bottles, sippy cups, the dental sealant in our mouths, plastic knives, forks and spoons, food storage containers—the list is nearly endless.

Polycarbonate is made from Bisphenol A. It comprises the epoxy resins that line the inside of food containers and beverage cans. Small amounts of BPA leach out when the plastic or can lining containers come in contact with food or water. According to Michael Shelby of the National Institute of Environmental Health Sciences (NIEHS), a division of the National Institutes of Health in Research Triangle Park, North Carolina, nearly 100% of our BPA exposure occurs this way. "Low levels of BPA are also found in house dust, the air and in water," adds Shelby, who directs the NIEHS's center for the Evaluation of Risks to Human Reproduction.[5]

What worries some scientists is that BPA is an estrogenic "mimic" that activates the same receptors in the body as estrogen does. In fact, BPA was first studied in the 1930s as a synthetic estrogen for women. Hormones are the messengers in the body's endocrine system. Chemicals like BPA are called "endocrine disruptors." "BPA is the largest volume endocrine disrupting chemical in commerce," says BPA critic Frederick Vom Saul, a biologist at the University of Missouri. Worldwide, more than six million pounds of BPA are manufactured every year. Vom Saul is convinced that BPA causes a host of problems, including breast and prostate cancer.[6]

Exposure to BPA can occur from such common, everyday things as conventional foods, car exhaust, fingernail polish, hair and other aerosol sprays, paints, and the noxious vapor compounds released from carpets, wallpaper, and magazine ink. BPA from all of these can contribute to a congested liver, which can cause the body to manifest such visible markers as spider veins, hemorrhoids, varicose veins, skin tabs on the neck and around the body, and the elusive cherry hemangiomas. If any of these appear on your body or those of any family members, it may be time to evaluate what you are doing to protect yourselves from toxic exposure.

Studies show that canned foods are a common source of daily BPA exposure in our lives. Cans of soda generally contain less BPA than canned pasta or soup! The worst foods tested contain enough BPA to put pregnant women and formula-fed infants much closer to dangerous levels than the government typically allows. Even some liquid infant formula is packed in cans lined with BPA, which seems ludicrous given the special vulnerabilities of children's developing systems.[7]

But before you run out and buy a metal water bottle, make sure you know what you're getting. Many reusable metal water bottles are lined with the same BPA-leaching plastic found in cans of food. How do you get rid of it? Unfortunately, BPA is so widely used and manufactured that none of us are likely to eliminate it from our system altogether. So how do we minimize our exposure to BPA? Here are some practical tips:

- Avoid plastic containers made of polycarbonate. Any bottle or container made of polycarbonate on it has No. 7 on the bottom. But the No. 7 can also appear on plastics that don't contain BPA.

- When possible, prepare or store food—especially hot foods and liquids—in glass, porcelain, or stainless steel dishes or containers.

- If you have polycarbonate plastic containers, don't microwave them. The plastic is more likely to break down and release BPA when it is repeatedly heated at high temperatures.

- Don't wash polycarbonate containers in the dishwasher. The detergent may break down the plastic, which would release BPA.

- If you use infant bottles, get bottles that are made of glass or BPA-free plastic. Born Free (newbornfree.com) is one of the first

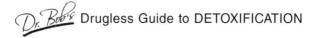

companies that make them. This is very important for the health of your children.

- When possible, replace canned foods with foods that are fresh, frozen, or packaged in aseptic (shelf stable) boxes. Be mindful and look for the words, "BPA-free."

- Avoid older versions of Delton dental sealant. Dental sealants are plastic resins that a dentist bonds into the grooves of the chewing surface of a tooth to help prevent cavities.

- When possible, and especially if you're pregnant and when feeding a young child, limit the amount of canned food in your diet.

- Avoid using old or scratched polycarbonate bottles. If you're in the market for a new water bottle, look for stainless steel water bottles that do not have a plastic liner.

- Soft or cloudy-colored plastic does not contain BPA. If you're formula feeding your infant, consider using powdered formulas packaged in non-steel cans.

Just Tell Me What to Do!

- Do not eat foods that have added colors. Focus on whole foods that are not packaged.

- Avoid partially hydrogenated or trans fat. Become label savvy. Read the Nutrition Facts Panel on the reverse side of the label and see if there are partially hydrogenated oils listed. If so, there is trans fat, but not enough per serving to be considered bad. I would not purchase that product.

- Use flax oil on your salads. Heat food with olive or rice oil. Avoid soy oils.

- Eliminate canned food that has plastic in the liners.

- Do not give your children sippy cups with the Number 7 on the bottom.

- Do not microwave food items covered or wrapped in plastic.

Endnotes

1. *Nutrition Action Newsletter*, Center for Science in the Public Interest, April 2008.

2. *Nutrition Action Newsletter*, Center for Science in the Public Interest, "Chemical Cuisine." May 2008.

3. The study was published online on March 26, 2007, and appeared in the April 10, 2007, print issue of *Circulation: Journal of the American Heart Association*.

4. Animal Studies Nutrition Action, Center for Science in the Public Interest, April 2008.

5. *Nutrition Action Newsletter*, Center for Science in the Public Interest, April 2008.

6. Ibid.

7. Ibid.

Chapter 3

WHAT YOU EAT BECOMES YOU!

Toxic substances in our food, drink, and general environment can disrupt the natural chemical and nutritional balance in our bodies, creating a state of toxicity that can impair proper and efficient organ function. This means that a toxic condition in the body overstresses the bodily organs, particularly those organs related to digestion and waste elimination—the colon, liver, kidneys, and stomach—because they have to work harder to metabolize the toxins and restore proper balance. Often they are unable to do so, because of excessive exposure resulting in a sustained state of toxicity, which can then lead to illness, including the complete or partial failure of the overtaxed organs. Dialysis, organ transplant, or other radical surgery commonly follows.

Understanding how body toxicity occurs—and taking appropriate action early—can go a long way in preventing such radical solutions, and even, in many cases, reversing damage that is already underway. As always, however, it is important to consider all detoxification protocols *in conjunction with* health care counsel and treatment provided by an experienced healthcare provider.

In this chapter we will examine the issue of toxicity with regard to the effect it has on the function and health of two major regulatory glands in the body: the hypothalamus and the thyroid. Both of these glands are part of our body's *endocrine system,* and have a major influence on whole body function.

The endocrine system regulates the body's major continuous and prolonged processes:

- Reproduction.

- Growth and development.

- Cellular metabolism and energy.

- Blood balance of nutrients, electrolytes, and water.

- Mobilization of body defenses against stressors (things that cause wear and tear on the body's physical and mental resources).

The endocrine system is made up of eight different glands located strategically throughout the body:

- The ovaries (or in men, the testes); source of progesterone and estrogen.

- Adrenals, located on top of the kidneys; these make sex, mineral regulating, and sugar balance hormones.

- Pancreas islets, part of the pancreas; creates insulin and enzymes.

- Thyroid, located in the throat; source of thyroid hormone.

- Para thyroid, part of the thyroid mechanism; assists in calcium function.

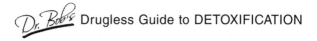

- Pineal, located in the brain, has control of how light affects the body.

- Pituitary, secretes many leading hormone activators.

- Hypothalamus, the "CEO" of the body, because it regulates and controls the others.

Besides these major organs, the endocrine system includes pockets of hormone-producing cells in tissues in the small intestines, heart, kidneys, and stomach. The endocrine system develops and begins producing hormones by the end of the second trimester of fetal development.

It is safe to say that the endocrine system is probably the first system impacted by nutritional imbalances and deficiencies. Viable nutrients are needed to make and replace hormones because the metabolic functions performed by hormones are nutrient based and mediated. Our bodies take what we give them and try to function optimally. However, our tissues, glands, and organs cannot operate properly with wrong or insufficient nutritional fuel any more than an automobile can operate with the wrong fuel in its tank.

The hypothalamus is the commander-in-chief of our hormonal system. I like to think of it as the maestro of the body. Just as a gifted musical maestro can take a collection of musicians who on their own sound great and guide them to blend together in an even more beautiful and emotionally moving symphony of sound, in a similar manner the hypothalamus connects the emotional and physical parts of our being. The hypothalamus controls autonomic reflexes such as the activity of the heart, digestive function, and the smooth muscles. One of its jobs is to connect your emotions to physical activity. You know that feeling you get in the pit of your stomach at times, along with loose stools. Your hypothalamus regulates function that you do not think about. It houses the body's thermostat as well as its biological clock, which maintains the body's rhythm of the 24-hour sleep/wake cycles. Sleep is necessary for your body to have the ability to clean itself up.

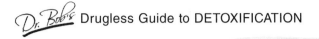

The hypothalamus is the commander-in-chief of our hormonal system.

In women, the hypothalamus also initiates the female cycle by producing the gonadotropin-releasing hormone (GnRH), which signals the pituitary to secrete the follicle-stimulating hormone (FSH). FSH stimulates the ovaries to secrete estrogen, the sex hormone that stimulates development of breast, uterine, and ovarian tissue. Synthetic Hormone Replacement Treatment (HRT) forms are associated with excessive cell growth that may lead to cancer. Females hormones need to be balanced so you do not have to take synthetic compounds that create unnecessary stress to the detoxifying components. Your body processes medications so they are less harmful to be eliminated.

When estrogen reaches a certain level, it signals the hypothalamus to trigger the pituitary to secrete the lutenizing hormone (LH). Estrogen levels then fall, while the level of LH rises and peaks (around day 14 of the 28-day cycle), stimulating ovulation, the release of an egg from its ovarian follicle. After ovulation, the follicle (now called the corpus luteum) is filled with cholesterol, which is first converted to pregnenolone (a hormone precursor) and then to progesterone. The newly made progesterone is used, in part, for the building up of the uterine lining. If after about 13 to 15 days the egg is not fertilized, the uterine lining is sloughed off in menstruation, when both estrogen and progesterone levels drop. Both estrogen and progesterone are necessary in the female cycle, and their *balance is key for full health!*

Many women in our Western culture have an imbalance of these hormones, especially insufficient levels of progesterone to counter excessive estrogen—*an imbalance that is further complicated by chronic stress, liver congestion*, and low levels of iodine, resulting in a poorly functioning thyroid and ovaries. You can see how important the liver is. It is necessary to metabolize hormonal function.

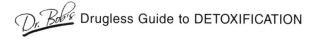

Progesterone, which is derived from a precursor steroid called pregnenolone, is important for a number of body functions. During times of stress or conditions of chronic adrenal hyper-stimulation, pregnenelone is capable of being converted into progesterone and then to the stress hormone cortisol (natural cortisone, which helps takes away pain and affects blood sugar stress). This explains why both men and women go to their healthcare provider tired and in pain, only to find out that their cholesterol is high. Cholesterol is a precursor to natural cortisone. Bodies taxed by stress and excessive inflammation tend to overcompensate by producing too much cholesterol.

Persistent and prolonged stress, which is so common in our day, is also a significant contributor to a toxic condition in the body. When someone goes through chronic stress or severe long-term stress, the hypothalamus will at first trigger an over production of the adrenal hormones, especially cortisol and dehydroepiandrosterone (DHEA). This eventually leads to adrenal weakness, a state in which the exhausted adrenals cannot respond adequately. Common symptoms include chronic tiredness, sensitivity to bright light, a craving for carbohydrates and salt, low blood pressure, and chronic back trouble.

Food cravings resulting from stress become an insidious negative feedback that causes people to become addicted to food that perpetuate additional stress to the organs responsible for your survival and elimination.

One very damaging adrenal dysfunction is excessive cortisol production, which causes, among other serious problems, increased calcium mobilization from the bones, leading to osteoporosis or loss of bone density. In a person with a healthy stress response, excessive levels of cortisol are automatically buffered. Constant stress destroys this feedback loop.

Hormonal imbalances compromise not only physical health but also psychological health, manifesting as problems ranging from depression to panic disorder. One way the body tries to compensate for imbalances created and exacerbated by the demands of stress is to overproduce key hormones. Another way

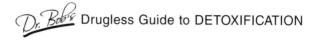

it tries to compensate is by converting sex hormones to stress hormones, thus further diminishing reproductive functions and the enjoyment of sexual health. This, by far, is one of the leading body signals that I see in my practice—the loss of sexual desire. If you do not have the desire or ability to engage in sexual intimacy, you probably have a severely drained system that needs to be recharged. This is very common in today's busy, often dual-income families, with our overcommitted lives, trying to balance between family, work, church, and extracurricular activities. *You can have emotional toxicity, which affects the liver.* When someone is angry for whatever reason, my experience suggests once again that the liver is impacted. Body signals include bloating a few hours after eating.

The Thyroid Keeps the Body Going

The thyroid is also adversely affected by chronic stress, as well as by the presence of toxic substances taken in from outside the body. This gland's role includes regulating calcium metabolism. Under normal conditions, the fight or flight response from adrenal stimulation causes the thyroid to increase glucose breakdown. Glucose is the fuel to the system.

In conditions of chronic stress or inflammation, however, the thyroid becomes overstimulated and eventually becomes depleted. Some of the signals of low thyroid function include cold hands and feet, hot flashes, depression, *constipation*, thinning hair, morning headaches, thinning outside eyebrows, wide-spaced teeth, sluggishness, high cholesterol, and menstrual problems, including scanty menses. Excessive estrogen also disrupts thyroid function, but this can be prevented by adequate progesterone levels.

In recent years both hyperthyroidism (overactive thyroid functioning) and especially hypothyroidism (low functioning) have become more common than they once were. Although there are many causal factors for this increase, the roles of nutrition, diet, and body toxification are too significant to be ignored.

If the body becomes toxic because of consuming the wrong kinds of foods, this may
inhibit the thyroid's ability to manufacture
critical hormones. Poor diet selections and toxicity in the body may lead to a deficiency in
tyrosine (an amino acid or protein building
block) and iodine, both of which are necessary
for proper thyroid function. When the thyroid
is not up to par or optimal function, you will
experience fatigue and reduced energy.
Constipation is also a common challenge and
major factor in toxic build up. The thyroid is
very important to keep the colon moving.

Tyrosine deficiency has been identified as
one causal link to depression, which is occur-
ring at record levels today, especially among
teenagers and children. The pattern for this
breakdown of physiology resulting in emotional burnout often begins at birth. A baby
who is bottle fed with soy-based formula from
the beginning, rather than breast fed, likely
faces potential health challenges in later years.
The soy found in baby formula is an anti-thy-
roid food. It has been my observation that children who are not breast fed are more than

likely consuming food that impairs thyroid function, and this from the beginning of life!

People of all ages today face increased depression issues in part because of their food choices. The current generation of young adults was raised by parents who were exposed to convenience foods in their early lives. This means that today's moms ate fries and chicken nuggets and the like during their formative years and have since had babies who have now grown up and are in their late teens and early twenties. Convenience and fast food are fried in or are overloaded with unhealthy oils that do not make good hormone precursors. The thyroid gland, like other glands in the endocrine system, depends on healthy oil as a basis to make the precious hormone keys for the body to function.

Convenience and fast food are fried in or are overloaded with unhealthy oils.

One of the biggest issues with thyroid dysfunction is a deficiency in iodine. Iodine is a

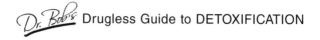

halide. On the periodic chart in chemistry you will notice it is in the same row as fluorine, bromine, and chlorine. These are antagonistic to iodine. If you are consistently exposed to these halides via unfiltered municipal water, dishwasher detergents, toothpastes and mouth washes, and select beverage and white bread that have bromine in it, or if you swim or exercise in a pool or hot tub, it is possible you can be overloaded with chemicals that will sabotage thyroid function. You want your thyroid at par, because it has everything to do with metabolism and elimination. It keeps the heat up.

An additional factor is focusing too much on carbohydrates and not enough on proteins. Toss in the fact that most of the protein consumed by most people comes from an inadequate source, usually refined, processed "pseudo-meat" such as chicken nuggets, sausage, and much deli meat. Protein from a qualified, natural, whole source is needed for L-Tyrosine.

As mentioned in the previous chapter, the public has been so focused on the low fat diet that the thought of allowing even a drop of good oil to pass their lips would be tantamount to taking poison. Actually, the opposite is true! The poison is actually the trans fat and other artificial additives they take in their sincere effort to avoid "bad" fat. The general population believes that all oil is bad, so now they primarily eat low fat, high carbohydrate foods. Consequently, the thyroid does not have the proper oil it needs. When the thyroid is unable to function properly, it causes the body to run on low with no energy and the system just dragging along. One of the ultimate consequences is weight gain and sluggish colon activity. *When the colon is sluggish, it creates compensatory stress to the liver.*

For most people the solution is simple: eat whole foods with a proper balance of protein and minerals.

In very simple terms, here is how the thyroid operates. Thyroid function is significant for normal bowel movements as mentioned

previously and is an indicator of iodine suffi-
ciency. Insufficient iodine in the thyroid means
insufficient iodine in the ovaries or testes,
which can negatively affect reproductive
health and function.

The thyroid gland is a small mass of tissue,
normally weighing less than one ounce,
located in the front of the neck, just below the
larynx. It is made up of two halves, called
lobes, that lie along the windpipe (trachea)
and are joined together by a narrow band of
thyroid tissue, known as the isthmus. During
development (inside the womb) the thyroid
gland originates in the back of the tongue, but
it normally migrates to the front of the neck
before birth. Sometimes it fails to migrate
properly and is located high in the neck or
even in the back of the tongue (lingual thyroid), which is very rare. At other times it may
migrate too far and ends up in the chest, which
is also rare.

The function of the thyroid gland is to
take iodine, found in many foods, and con-
vert it into thyroid hormones, thyroxine (T4)

and triiodothyronine (T3). Thyroid tissue cells combine iodine and the amino acid, tyrosine, to make T3 and T4, which are then released into the bloodstream and transported throughout the body, where they control metabolism (conversion of oxygen and calories to energy). Every cell in the body depends upon thyroid hormones for regulation of their metabolism. The normal thyroid gland produces about 80 percent T4 and about 20 percent T3. However, T3 possesses about four times the hormone "strength" of T4.

The thyroid gland is under the control of the pituitary gland, a small gland the size of a peanut located at the base of the brain. When the level of thyroid hormones drops too low, the pituitary gland produces Thyroid Stimulating Hormone (TSH), which stimulates the thyroid gland to produce more hormones. Under the influence of TSH, the thyroid will manufacture and secrete T3 and T4, thereby raising their blood levels. The pituitary senses this and responds by decreasing its TSH production. Imagine the thyroid

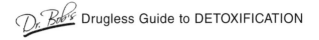

gland as a furnace and the pituitary gland as the thermostat. Thyroid hormones are like heat. When the heat gets back to the thermostat, it turns the thermostat off. As the room cools (the thyroid hormone levels drop), the thermostat turns back on (TSH increases) and the furnace produces more heat (thyroid hormones).

Like all other glands of the endocrine system, the pituitary gland is regulated by the hypothalamus. The hypothalamus is part of the brain and produces TSH, which tells the pituitary gland to stimulate the thyroid gland (release TSH). One might imagine the hypothalamus as the person who regulates the thermostat since it tells the pituitary gland at what level the thyroid should be set.

In addition to widespread "fat phobia," our society also suffers from an epidemic of "iodine phobia," where little emphasis is being placed on supplementation with an organic source of iodine. For most people, iodized table salt is the primary source of additional iodine, but it is not the best-quality source.

Commercial-grade sodium chloride also has anti-caking constituents, including aluminum and dextrose (or sugar), which are included so the table salt will flow uninterrupted.

Salt Phobia

"Salt phobia" is also a major problem today. People have been advised to avoid salt because it raises blood pressure. In my own practice I have found that salt may raise blood pressure in about 5 percent of patients, and this from sodium chloride, common commercial-grade table salt. More significant to increased blood pressure, in my experience, is our insatiable appetite for sweets. Sugar raises the insulin level in the body and stresses the adrenal gland, raising blood pressure. The body compensates with increased sodium retention. Increased sodium retention creates increased water retention. I also see blood pressure elevation in patients who do not drink enough water. When someone does not drink enough water, the blood gets thicker and more concentrated, restricting the flow. That is why it is important to drink at least one quart of pure water daily, minimum.

Rather than common table salt, which I never use, I recommend Celtic Sea Salt®, which is harvested from the northern coast of France. Nothing has been added to it. The granules come from the open rock surface where the salt has evaporated from ocean water. It should be called Celtic Sea Minerals instead of Sea Salt. Celtic Sea Salt is an excellent source of minerals, and I encourage our patients to use it liberally.

The key to repair of thyroid function is restoring hormonal balance through supplementation from pure, natural sources. Just as with insulin from a cow for diabetics, thyroid hormones from an outside source does not repair the gland; it merely controls the symptoms.

I often suggest taking nutritional supplementation designed to feed the various glands the nutrients needed to restore cellular function.

If, after consulting with a healthcare professional, you decide to take an iodine supplement, go slowly. At first you may notice a skin rash, a metallic taste in your mouth, and/or pain over the eyes. Keep in mind also that taking any supplement, whether it is natural or synthetic, can interfere with some medications. And some individuals have symptoms that appear to indicate they are sensitive to iodine. **Your body is adapting to the release of the toxic effects of fluorine, chlorine, and bromine that are being displaced by iodine.** These symptoms should go away in a few days. Patients on heart medication may notice heartbeat alterations when taking iodine. For these reasons, *always talk to a knowledgeable healthcare professional before beginning these protocols.* Do not attempt to take large doses of iodine on your own when you are taking Amiodarone, Pacerone, or Cardarone.

Japanese women, who traditionally have minimal menopause symptoms or hot flashes, consume up to 12 mg of iodine a day in their food, normally from fish and sea vegetables. Having spent extended time in Japan,

I know firsthand that sea vegetables and fresh marine life are major staples of their diet. Also, the Japanese traditionally eat as a family, so it is rare to see them eating at fast food chains as we do in our Western culture. Their markets overflow with fresh fish that is available daily.

Dietary Journals

I also like to see my patients' dietary journals to make sure they are eating adequate protein. Most Americans today do not consume enough protein, for example, chicken, turkey, lamb, and yes, even periodic red meat. Because of this, I encourage my patients to eat at least three to five ounces of organic-sourced protein with each meal.

To be sure, understanding the nature and causes of body toxicity can be a complex and even intimidating exercise. The good news: correcting the problem and detoxifying your body is usually not so complicated. It is a matter of following some simple protocols and using common sense regarding diet and exercise. The human body has a tremendous God-given ability to heal itself. Oftentimes all it needs is the opportunity.

Detoxification, essentially, is nothing more than giving the body the opportunity to heal itself. Now it is time to take the first step to a healthier you.

Just Tell Me What to Do!

- Eat whole foods. They feed the hormonal system. Avoid processed foods whenever possible. Do not eat fried foods—ever!

- I would suggest you look into green detergents. Avoid chlorine dishwashing detergents. These items are toxic to your thyroid.

- Find a source of sea vegetables, commonly found in most health food stores. Kelp supplements are a good supplement and source of iodine. Celtic Sea Salt can be used as a source of iodine.

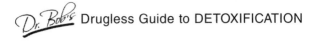

- Be aware of your exposure to chlorine, flu-orine, and bromine. You may want to pur-chase a shower de-chlorinator.

- Eat organic protein. I encourage three to five ounces with each meal. Avoid soy, it is antagonistic to the thyroid function.

- Journal what you are eating for a week or two. Use the template in the Appendix and jot down your meals. You may be surprised at how much you eat. A good percentage of all meals are eaten out of the home, with-out knowing the ingredients.

Let's Talk About the Lymphatic System

The lymphatic system is probably one of the most mysterious systems in the body. You only really hear about it from an exercising rebounder enthusiast that bounces daily to get the clear lymphatic fluid moving, or unfortu-nately from the cancer patient who has been advised by their physician that the cancer has spread to the lymph nodes. The oncologist (cancer physician) usually says something to the effect, "It appears that the chemotherapy and radiation only contained the cancer for awhile." Heart-wrenching words echo through the cortex of your brain.

I will introduce you to the mechanics of the lymphatic system. It would be to your best interest to take care of it like you would the down spouts on your home, the drain in your bath tub or shower, and the road gutter in front of your house. *The lymphatic system is a network of multi-tasked channels.* It is literally your body's sewer system—one of several lines of defense of your immune system, and the freight train hauling around fuel in the form of food particles. It is like the "patriot missile" line of defense, the infantry and sup-ply chain all in one package.

The lymphatic system is part of the defense mechanism in the body. It activates lymphocytes and carries proteins and fats for digestion. The nodes in a person's neck, including the tonsils, swell and get red when they are protecting you. Having your tonsils removed is like disarming a warrior or cutting

the wire to the "warning signal" on your dash-
board.

**When we are born there should be little tags
on all of our organs that say:
DO NOT REMOVE.**

We have been told that commonly
removed organs are not necessary to live. I
believe as time goes on we will hear more and
more about the negative effects of the surgical
removal of lymph tissue. *The tonsils are the storage house mechanism of sulfur in the body.* Sulfur
is needed to help make cartilage for your
structural health. Have you ever wondered
why so many people are taking chondroitin
sulfated products? They take it for the sulfur.
Great natural sources of sulfur include eggs,
onion, and garlic. If your lymph nodes are
swollen and sore; limit dairy, exercise your
muscles, and drink more water. It is very
important to understand that when these and
other tissues in your body are doing their job,
you *should not remove them!*

You need to assess why your lymph nodes are swollen and sore. Usually it is from consuming something that is overworking the system. If you continue the behavior long enough, the result is some type of chronic condition—including *cancer*. Your children are no different; if they continually have swollen glands *don't give them another antibiotic. Stop feeding them sugar and dairy products.* I also encourage lymphatic drainage massage by an experienced massage therapist. This assists your body's line of defense and creates opening drainage for toxins that have accumulated in your tissues.

The word *stagnant* should be part of your wellness vocabulary. *When the lymphatic system is **stagnant** your body is not working at 100 percent.* It is important to keep all the fluids in your body moving at a nice rate, with no congestion or bottle necks. Several of the primary reasons I see sluggish or stagnant lymphatic systems is because the person is eating too much dairy, not drinking enough water, and lack of muscle-moving exercise. *Motion is life.* It is easier to move clear lymphatic fluid versus the sludge created by a no-water, soda (diet soda included), power drink (loaded with chemicals), alcohol, and coffee diet.

The cells in your body are like machines, all working together for the good of the whole. When a machine is operating, there is generally some scrap or waste from the manufacturing operation. The maintenance crew commonly comes by and picks it up for the recycle bin. There is waste or a by-product of production. Your cells have waste, and part of the waste disposal system is your lymphatic channels in and around your arms, legs, neck, trunk, and abdomen. Wastes are eventually processed by the liver, kidneys, and colon for recycling or elimination. Your colon has one of the largest concentrations of lymphatic tissue.

The lymphatic system also creates the warriors or lymphocytes that seek and destroy foreign invaders or cells that have become abnormal. The lymphatic system is like the maintenance crew sweeping, cleaning, and disposing—it is capable of handling only so much at a time. If the channels used to carry away the material are congested from overproduction or faulty disposal, it can get backed up.

This reaction can be compared to when there is an abnormally large amount of rain. The gutters on a house and down spouts can handle only so much rainfall in a limited time period. If you fail to clean the gutters, accumulated leaves and sludge can cause trouble, including water damage inside the house and overflow into the basement. I know from experience that this can happen.

You may have a sump pump in your basement. The way the foundations are generally designed, all of the roof run-off water makes its way into the basement sump hole crock. A 4 to 6-inch pipe spews the water in, and one or two pumps expel the water to the main sewer in the street. Note: if you have 4 inches of pipe coming in, it is best to have at least 4 inches going out. Why? Because if you have too much coming in and not enough going out, your basement will flood.

If you have two pumps working very diligently during a downpour, you are probably feeling good about the situation. But all of a sudden you hear a crack of lightning and the power goes off. If you did not plan ahead with a battery backup pump or gas-powered generator, you may end up with a huge mess in the basement.

The outcome of both scenarios can be controlled. Although you cannot control the amount of rain, you can control how the water is disposed. Your body is no different. You cannot necessarily control everything that is thrown at your body, but you do have charge over what you do with it. (And honestly you really do have control of the majority of what goes in, even the level of toxins. You can relocate if there is a serious health issue.) Let me explain.

First, make sure you are drinking enough water every day. How much is enough? Well, the least amount you should drink is a quart. A general rule of thumb is to drink one ounce of water for every pound of body weight. I personally would not drink more than 100 ounces a day, especially if you start noticing leg cramps at night or when you are walking. You lose too many minerals if you drink too much water. As I mentioned before and this is important: *avoid drinking soda, fruit drinks, energy drinks, or coffee as your main beverage.* Eat veggies and fruits; they have high water content. Avoid pastries and goodies that draw water out of the system to be processed.

Your colon is a dehydrator, if you eat wheat-based items you can create coverings on intestinal walls that are thick and pasty. Your body needs water to cleanse the system. The next time you are hungry, instead of grabbing a "little" piece of cracker or cookie, drink a glass of water or eat a piece of cucumber, small tomato, or piece of celery. You are putting fluid in your body that is positively proactive for your long-term health, instead of creating a negative state.

Make sure you are exercising regularly. A rebounder (small mini-trampoline) works physiologically by creating a vacuum in the

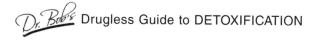

lymphatic channels. This creates movement of fluid. *Motion is life.* Any type of exercise is better than being a couch potato. Walking, riding a bike, fast-stepping, dancing, any type of motion. Your lymphatic system does not have the privilege of having its own pump like the cardiovascular system does—you must *move* to make it work properly.

Several massage therapists assist me in my clinical setting; and they complete therapeutic massage treatments. One of the techniques that they have all specialized in is lymphatic drainage massage. I have recommended patients for this massage who have swelling in their bodies; they have seen this swelling diminish by having their lymphatic system properly stimulated and drained.

I recently presented a workshop on skin health. When I commented that the average Western female absorbs, through friction or natural lip-licking, up to 4 to 7 pounds of lipstick over their lifetime, a massage therapist in attendance said she has noticed that when a female patient with lipstick on has a lymphatic massage the lipstick or gloss is absorbed. She theorized that she was stimulating the flow of lymph fluid in the body. I thought that was a very interesting observation that I had not read or heard of.

Most people who have dry lips don't realize that the problem is internal. Dry lips are a possible signal that you may need to increase your water consumption. Most would not think of the lips as a tissue directly linked to the lymph channels. If you are a massage therapist and you do lymphatic drainage, observe that phenomenon and let me know if you see the same thing.

The lymphatic system is not the "bad guy"— it is critical for your optimal health. For optimal health, your objective is to keep the lymph channels flowing flawlessly. I generally observe the following case history. The patient has a long history of poor diet choices; I have seen this thousands of times when I review the food journals of my patients. Consumption choices are usually focused on food that does not promote regular, timely,

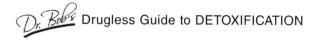

no-assistance-needed bowel movements (that means without a laxative, natural herb, or otherwise), and are mostly concentrated on refined grains and starches. *These people have toxic-looking skin, which is pale, not pink and vibrant, with many brown marks, and varicose and spider veins.* Little or no exercise is common in the intake history. All of these factors result in a stagnant system trying to get rid of the excess scrap from production.

The body is overwhelmed; it does not know what to do with all the excess. The environment in the body is at a point of what a toxic pond or river would look like. Cells begin to break down; there is cell membrane destruction, a condition called oxidation which is like massive rusting away occurs. You can slow and stop the oxidation process, which is like the deterioration progression of steel, by increasing your consumption of veggies during the day. Vegetables and fruits are like Rustoleum and combine with the "free radicals" theorized to be in the process.

The tremendous magnitude of oxidation creates the potential for free radical or abnormal cell activity; hormonal levels are anything but normal. For women, for some time they don't "feel good," and then symptoms may appear; a lump on the breast, menses is heavy, and a feeling of nausea. When you finally go to the doctor; many tests are completed and then you have the consultation when you are told you have *cancer*.

You make an appointment for further testing with a cancer specialist who decides to do a biopsy. You wait with baited breath for the results, you are receiving well-wishes from friends and family, e-mails from people with advice about what to do, and finally you are told the cancer has spread to your lymphatic system. They want to take the nodes out—so now what do you do?

Here is my advice to my patients. This is what I say every time, as diplomatically as possible. "If you don't change what you are doing you will DIE!" That usually gets their attention, with a tear. I am not trying to be abrasive. We are in a battle. You are the commander and chief of your army, what you decide to do affects the *victory*. You need to take responsibility to fight your own war. *What you have done to this point in your life is the reason you are in your situation.*

The big question: what about the chemotherapy and radiation treatment? My suggestions: Ask yourself how bad your symptoms are. What stage is the cancer? Sometimes, if the cancer is advanced, you may need the extra help to get it under control while you are making lifestyle changes. If your cancer is not advanced, then you have a fighting chance to win the war. I see cases like this all the time in my natural, drugless practice. *I have had new patients present themselves to the office with a tear in the eye, make the decision to* **change,** *and they* **live.** I do not heal them, their own body does the healing; I coach them. Unfortunately many come in when the conventional methods have been exhausted, and there is nothing else they can do; hardly a time to start thinking about making lifestyle changes.

Very honestly, and this is not meant to disparage the established ways, *chemotherapy and radiation are not the **only** answers—they do not get to the cause of the problem.* They only treat the symptoms. **Clean machines work better.** You need to clean the machine. Synthetic Hormone Replacement Treatment (HRT) for female hormonal issues was the standard treatment by the medical community, but women were dying because of synthetically sourced "horse urine"-based medication. Drugging females would have continued, had it not been for the extremely significant results of a government study released in 2003. It is important to realize **the battle you are in is to save your life.**

Just Tell Me What to Do!

* Focus on whole foods that promote bowel movement. Mixed greens and mostly raw (lunch) and steamed (dinner) vegetables should be a regular part of your diet.

* Drink water as your beverage of choice. Avoid dairy, which tends to plug the lym-

phatic channels. Eating cheese on a regular basis, according to the senior massage therapist on staff at my office, creates a layer of palpable fat under the skin. Her clients who are regular cheese consumers have a peculiar odor to their skin and especially their feet.

- Exercise your muscles regularly—that means *every day*. Bounce on a large 55cm exercise ball or mini-trampoline.

- Stretch your muscles with flexibility exercises using a band.

- Tonsils removed? Eat eggs, onion, and garlic. An organic egg a day is safe and good for you. Eat the yolk. Make it poached, hard boiled, or scrambled with olive oil. Put some spinach in the egg, with the onions and, what the heck, put in a dash of garlic. No need to have toast.

- Eat Dr. Bob's ABCs every day. One-half of a sweet apple, several pieces of baked or grated raw beets, and several small organic baby carrots or a large carrot that has been peeled and cut into bite-size pieces. (See Appendix D, Detoxification Food Selection and Consumption.)

- Start your day with a quarter wedge of an organic lemon in pure warm or hot water. This is good for the liver and digestion.

- Eliminate the consumption of soda and alcohol, and limit coffee consumption. Soda has manmade chemicals that stress the liver and kidneys. Alcohol, including wine, even in moderation still needs to be processed. Some of today's literature says alcohol will help your heart, but this isn't always true.

- Eliminating deserts and wine with your meals promotes a more healthy life. It has been my experience that patients who have the discipline to curtail alcohol, lose weight, and lower their cholesterol overcome depression more quickly than those who hold to the "moderation" theory.

Chapter 4

DETOXIFICATION ACTION STEPS

By now you may be thinking, *OK, Dr. Bob, I realize that my body is full of toxins and needs to be cleansed. What do I do now? How do I detoxify? There are so many things to consider that I feel overwhelmed by the challenge. Where do I start?*

Excellent questions. The issues of body toxicity and cleansing/purification may indeed seem overwhelming at first, especially for those just becoming familiar with this area of therapy. Don't despair; the answers are not as difficult or as complicated as you might think. The human body has an amazing capacity to heal itself; all it needs (usually) is the opportunity.

Detoxification is essentially a twofold process:

1. Learning how to avoid putting new toxins into the body.

2. Taking a few simple steps to help the body flush out existing toxins, thus giving the body the chance to heal itself.

So let's talk about cleansing.

Some Basic Protocols for Body Cleansing (Detoxification)

Simply stated, body cleansing, or detoxification, involves a change in dietary philosophy and practice. The goal is not a "quick fix" but lifestyle modification. Just as toxicity occurs from eating and drinking the wrong things, detoxification is achieved by learning to eat and drink the right things. Body cleansing promotes health and healing. It's not about taking more toxic medications but about making dietary changes and corrections so the body can heal itself.

Detoxification is achieved by learning to eat and drink the right things.

The detoxification process centers on cleansing the major organs of digestion and elimination: the liver, kidneys, and colon. In brief, common protocols for detoxification include cleansing herbs, juice or water fasting, whole food or raw diets, and colonic irrigation and hydrotherapy (sauna, steam, baths, soaks), liver herbs, and roots.

Cleansing herbs. Milk thistle, dandelion root/leaf, and yellow dock, for example, are great for cleansing the liver, while dandelion root works wonders for the kidneys. Yellow dock is also a great natural source of iron, making it of significant benefit to people with iron deficiencies. These liver-cleansing herbs are helpful also for young people, for whom the raging hormones of adolescence and puberty can often lead to a congested liver. For detailed information about herbs and their uses, see Appendix A.

Juice or water fasting. Done correctly and wisely, liquid fasts can be of benefit, but usually should be employed sparingly. The primary danger of a liquid fast is the risk of not consuming enough protein to maintain good muscle health. On the other hand, a juicing protocol can be extremely helpful for people with cancer or as a preventative measure against cancer. *I must stress, however, that such a juicing protocol should be used as a **supplement** to other cancer and anti-cancer treatments and protocols, **not** as a **substitute**!*

The juicing protocol I encourage for my patients is to drink at least one fresh quart of vegetable juice daily for a minimum of two months. The juice is to be made in eight-ounce increments and to be consumed immediately. I suggest the following items in the recipe: carrot, beet, ginger (small piece), sweet apple, parsley, celery, and cucumber. If desired, turmeric can be substituted for the ginger. Please watch the ingredients in the green food, and avoid any artificial sweeteners. I encourage my patients to focus on eating fresh veggies, avoiding all processed products and beverages.

For more information on juicing go to www.vitamix.com.

This combination assists the body in purifying itself and also significantly assists in the alkalizing process of the system. Acid promotes cancer and alkaline promotes life. Optimal health calls for our system to be slightly alkaline rather than acidic.

Whole food or raw diets rotated with steamed vegetables. Get in the habit of eating whole foods raw whenever possible. Organic foods are the best. Eating whole, raw, and organic ensures the fullest intake of essential nutrients, fiber, protein, and minerals. You can alternate steamed veggies and lightly sautéed veggies with olive as a viable alternative to raw. Some may have a challenge with raw only. Broccoli becomes vibrant green when heat is added, versus the dull hue of raw.

Colonic irrigation and hydrotherapy (sauna, steam, baths, soaks). Colonic irrigation is a special procedure that completely cleanses the colon. While from my experience it is not

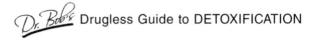

unsafe, it should be performed by a trained specialist. Don't try it at home by yourself.

A healthy colon is essential for a healthy body. Conventional diets comprised of refined, processed foods high in saturated fats and low in fiber contribute to many problems associated with the large intestine. The elimination of undigested food material and other waste products is as important as the digestion and assimilation of foodstuffs. Waste material allowed to remain stagnant in the colon results in decomposition of these substances and increased bacteria and their toxins.

The colon contains the largest concentration of bacteria in the body. These bacteria provide important functions, such as the synthesis of folic acid, B-vitamins, and vitamin K from foods. Bacillus coli and acidophilus comprise the majority of the healthy thousands of different kinds of bacteria in the colon, along with other disease-producing bacteria in small numbers. Waste material allowed to stagnate alters the proportion of healthy bacteria to disease-producing bacteria, and the potential for disease exists. These bacteria decompose proteins and carbohydrates, resulting in the production of toxins. Some of the toxins are thought to be absorbed and may be a potential source of disease elsewhere in the body.

The purpose of the colon as an eliminative organ is to remove this waste material by mass muscular contraction, called peristalsis. Colon hydrotherapy provides therapeutic improvement of muscular tone, facilitating peristalsis and benefiting the atonic (sluggish) colon. **Commonly precipitated by a sluggish thyroid, the effects of a stagnant colon can be manifested in the form of constipation, halitosis (bad breath), skin blemishes, headaches, low back pain, and lack of energy.**

I generally recommend two colonic irrigations per year, one in the fall (before Thanksgiving) and one in the spring (before Memorial Day).

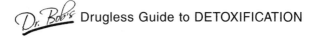

Focus on Foods that Support Elimination

The most common element of most detoxification programs is simply to eat less and focus on foods that support elimination. In other words, focus on vegetables and water versus refined pastries and chemically based beverages. And if possible, go organic with the vegetables, because organic food is free of highly toxic fungicides.

Cleansing programs are designed to be short-term, not prolonged protocols. It is not a logical strategy to eat anything you want with reckless abandon and then take a cleansing protocol to detoxify just so you can go back to your old bad habits. Cleansing protocols help remove toxins and give the body the chance to heal itself, but your long-term goal is to learn to eat "slow food" instead of "fast food."

Start planning ahead. Eat whole real food, and try to avoid genetically modified food items (GMO). The best way to do this is to eat organic foods. Some might think that is an extreme measure, but the less stress you put on your body, including your organs of digestion and elimination, the better. In nature all foods are designed to replace themselves.

An apple a day keeps the doctor away.

You've heard the old adage, "An apple a day keeps the doctor away." There is a lot of truth in that statement. Reactive oxidative species (ROS) is a normal part of cell metabolism that produces by-products that help kill disease-causing bacteria. If this process accelerates too rapidly, however, cell alteration or damage can result. Toxins accelerate the rate of ROS, while apples slow it down. According to the American Cancer Society, the number one cause of cancer is the genetic alteration of cell membranes.[1]

What causes this? An acceleration of toxins. A simple, healthy way to help keep oxidative reaction under control is to eat at least half an apple every day, preferably not green apples, but red ones such as Fuji, Gala, and

Delicious. Green apples, such as Granny Smith, can stagnate digestion.

It's All About the Liver

The primary function of the liver is to assist the body in absorbing what it needs and dumping out what it does not want. In other words, it aids the body in assimilation and digestion of essential nutrients as well as in the elimination of waste. Proper liver function, therefore, is essential to overall health. Some of the most important functions of the liver include:

- Metabolizing proteins, fats, and carbohydrates, thus providing energy and nutrients.

- Storing vitamins, minerals, and sugars

- Filtrating the blood and helping remove harmful chemicals and bacteria.

- Creating bile, which breaks down the fats.

- Helping to assimilate and store fat-soluble vitamins (A, D, E, K).

- Storing extra blood, which can be quickly released when needed.

- Creating serum proteins, which maintain fluid balance and act as carriers.

- Helping maintain electrolyte and water balance.

- Breaking down and eliminating excess hormones.

Toxins can come by eating fat-soluble foods through the food chain that have a natural affinity for fat-soluble membranes, such as livers. Conventional versus organic animal and fish tissue would be prime examples of this. This is why I recommend, as far as your budget will allow, that you eat organic meat. These fats can be stored for years and then released at times of low food intake, extra exercise, or stress. During these times you may experience flu-like symptoms, which may actually be your body dumping toxins.

The liver transforms the fat-soluble compounds into water-soluble substances to be excreted. This is one of the reasons why so many people have toxic tissues and body signals, such as spider veins and chronic body odor, nausea, hemorrhoids, bad breath, constipation, or diarrhea. All of these are body signals of a plugged or sluggish liver. When toxins are released by your body, you may experience symptoms such as tiredness, dizziness, nausea, a racing pulse, headaches, skin rash, or a heavy metal taste in your mouth.

The liver is also important in maintaining clean blood because it acts as a sort of blood filter. Herb "blood purifiers" that are often prescribed are not actually scrubbing the blood. What happens is that these herbs stimulate the blood flow through the liver, removing debris, old cells, and toxins. Also, they protect and stimulate the liver cells, encouraging the production of enzymes and helping to maintain a proper bowel chemical environment.

One common, low-tech, low-cost, but highly effective treatment for increasing blood flow that I recommend and use regularly with my patients is the Castor Oil Pack, used in conjunction with a heating pad. It has been used without side effects and is considered safe and normally can be used with great effect up to three times a week. If you are having liver issues I highly recommend it. Complete instructions for administering the Castor Oil Pack are found in Appendix B.

Liver herbs and roots. For many people, any discussion of herbs can become overwhelming very quickly because there are so many available. That's why I like to keep it as simple as possible. While there are many liver-healthy herbs, such as devil's claw, echinacea, feverfew, ginkgo, goldenseal, hawthorn, and marshmallow, I want to focus on the two primary ones I employ in my practice because they consistently bring the greatest results: milk thistle and dandelion root/leaf.

Milk thistle promotes milk secretion and is perfectly safe to be used by all breastfeeding mothers. It can also be used to increase the circulation and flow of bile from the liver and the gallbladder. Milk thistle contains a constituent called silymarin that protects liver cells from chemical damage.

Dandelion root/leaf is a bitter tonic for the liver that stimulates the activity of both liver and gallbladder function. This increases the flow of bile, which helps in constipation and indigestion. The leaves are powerful diuretics, and in contrast to drug diuretics, the herb does not leech potassium out of the body. This combination of liver and kidney effects make it a good cleansing remedy in skin and rheumatic problems.

Dandelion leaf is a great addition to your green salad. It helps purify the kidneys. Dandelion root supports healthy liver function. All it takes is five drops daily in your water.

For a more thorough discussion of herbs and their uses, see Appendix A.

A Word About Beets

In many ways the beet is the unsung hero of the vegetable world. Beet fiber lowers cholesterol.[2] The main effect is that it keeps fat from accumulating in the liver. If you have high triglycerides, beets will lower that because triglycerides are basically made of fat. According to Dr. Gina Nick in *Clinical Purification*, you could lower your cholesterol 40 percent by eating beets. Beets contain a high concentration of betaine, which has a methyl group in it that is useful in liver cleansing. Betaine also helps get rid of body stiffness, while betaine hydrochloride aids in digestion.

I generally recommend at least a third of a cup a day. I think the best way to prepare them is to grate them over a salad. Another good way to eat beets is to peel them, cut them up, add balsamic vinegar, olive oil, rice oil, coconut oil, or Celtic Sea Salt and cook them for an hour or until fork tender. Beets are part of "Dr. Bob's ABCs"—apples, beets, and carrots—each of which should be part of everyone's daily diet.

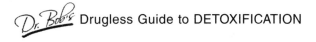

Gallbladder Issues

The gallbladder is analogous to a reservoir of emulsifying soap in the body, which is your whole body degreaser detergent, antioxidant, and source of alkaline ash. A lot of people today drink alkaline water. That's not really necessary. All you need to do is eat an apple a day to help keep your bowel moving which helps you stay alkaline balanced.

You want to keep the bile flowing, and that involves the gallbladder. As the regulator and storehouse for bile, the gallbladder is an essential organ for long-term health. Bile is extremely important because it emulsifies, or breaks down, fats from the large globules to the smaller ones that are more water-soluble. You do not want unprocessed large fats circulating in your body. When your gallbladder is removed, you in essence have lost proper fat metabolism in your body, which can precipitate heart problems. When your gallbladder has been removed, you have literally lost your reservoir of bile. Potentially your blood vessels will have more accumulated fatty deposits, and there is a greater possibility that you will develop blood vessel challenges. In such cases I recommend taking a whole food bile salt daily. Also, eating organic apples with the peel, applesauce freshly made by you, and organic are all helpful in improving bile flow.

Take a load off your liver...

Take a load off your liver by reducing fat and protein, especially dairy products, which are a major liver burden. Dairy is tough on the liver. If you experience digestive distress when you eat peanut butter, green peppers, onions, or cucumbers, it may be a sign of gallbladder distress. These foods may cause liver and gallbladder pain. If that is the case, make sure you drink more water. In addition, you may want to eat brown rice and millet and more vegetables like beets and others that do not cause distress.

Gallstones may interrupt normal bile flow. Bile flow can also be impaired by alcohol, thyroid dysfunction, some medications, synthetic high-potency, petro-chemically based vitamins like vitamin E, and the birth control pill. When your bile is stagnant, your skin may look yellow, sallow, or blemished. Also, important vitamins are not assimilated properly, which can impair blood clotting, vision, and the body's anti-oxidant system.

Peppermint leaf increases the flow of bile in your liver and gallbladder, making it a very important herb. Refer to Appendix E for more information about peppermint leaf.

How Does the Liver Detoxify?

How does the liver detoxify? Simply stated, the liver has a two-phase process. Phase one takes toxic substances from a fat-soluble state to water soluble, which is easier to eliminate. It does this by binding them or conjugating them with sulfur groups. This is one of the reasons I always encourage eggs, onions, garlic, beets, and cruciferous vegetables (cabbage, cauliflower, and broccoli). All these foods contain sulfur, which is necessary for detoxifying the body.

Your liver is obligated to assist you in getting rid of toxins. Phase two is also dependent on anti-oxidants, the levels of which are affected by your attitude and emotional state. So your liver can be affected not only by the foods you eat but also by the emotions you experience. Your endocrine glands, including the hypothalamus which connects your physical and emotional states, have a very significant association with your detoxification process.

The honest truth is that we are what we eat and drink.

So what can you do for the liver? First of all, you want to keep toxins to a minimum. The honest truth is that we are what we eat and drink. Either gender can have congestion or sluggishness in the body. Once again I recommend starting the day with a wedge of organic lemon in warm or hot water in the morning to stimulate liver function. Eat Dr. Bob's ABCs every day: apple (one-half), beets (one-third cup), and carrots (at least five baby carrots daily). Eat plenty of sulfur-based foods (eggs, onions, garlic, cabbage, cauliflower, and broccoli).

Avoid fried food, sugar, trans fat, and dairy. These are among the most common of all body toxins and are consumed in abundance. Take an assessment of your skin. If you have lesions, rashes, spider veins, or red cherry hemangioma skin tabs, these may be signs of liver stress. If you have had your gall-bladder removed, I recommend a whole food bile salt every day: one a day, two a day, three a day, and then back to one a day, repeating the cycle indefinitely. I also suggest the Castor Oil Pack (see Appendix B) at least once a week to promote liver function. (See also Appendix D, Detoxification Food Selection and Consumption.)

Skin Talk

Let's talk about skin for a bit more now that you have been shown the whole picture of how the body is interrelated. Blood purification also depends upon the proper function of all the elimination organs. The skin, for instance, eliminates large quantities of toxins through sweating. Sweating therapy increases the body's ability to throw off toxins. Drinking plenty of water can take a load off your liver. This is one reason why tea, coffee, fruit drinks, and alcohol can be an issue; they are diuretics. The main issue with fruit drinks is their high sugar content.

In my practice I have observed that people who sweat a lot often have adrenal gland exhaustion. The sympathetic nervous system has been used to capacity. Under normal function, the adrenal gland helps constrict blood vessels inside the body. When the adrenal gland does not have the ability to do this, another system takes over, called the parasympathetic nervous system. When this system takes over, the result is profuse sweating. An imbalance between these two systems can lead to excessive and unhealthy water loss. Drinking plenty of water is critical for hydrating the system and helping with cleansing.

Another area to be aware of is the lymphatic system, which was discussed in detail in a previous chapter. Tiny lymph channels that are connected to the skin absorb whatever is placed or rubbed onto the skin, where it is transported to larger lymph channels, which dump it into the veins, which take it to the liver, where it must be processed. Be careful—many of the commercial skin products available today are toxic.

One way to detoxify and stimulate the lymphatic system is through the use of a lymph brush, found at most health food stores. Start brushing from the feet and lower legs upward to the thighs, and then do the same with the arms. This will help move lymph fluids. Unlike the circulatory system, which has the heart to pump blood, the lymphatic system has no pump. For this reason, one of the things I recommend is to stimulate lymph fluid movement by bouncing on a large ball or a mini-trampoline for a few minutes each day.

Psoriasis, acne, and any other skin lesions can almost always be traced to congestion in the liver. The skin is a report card of what's going inside the body. Taking antibiotics to destroy intestinal bacteria will help acne over the short term, but in the long haul they can cause more challenges. As I said before, avoid dairy products because they overstress the liver. Reduce your consumption of wheat because wheat can also cause toxins to accumulate in the walls of your intestines.

Carrots can help the skin because of the precursors it contains to create vitamin A. What else can you do for the skin? Drink more water, consume less dairy, and eat apples, beets, and carrots every day. As a result, your bowels will start to move better, your body will absorb fewer toxins, and your skin will clear up.

One final note on the liver: to improve liver and gallbladder function, particularly if you show signs of sluggish or impaired function, you may want to consider a liver/gallbladder flush. This is an easy and effective way to clean out the bile ducts, accelerate elimination of toxins, and allow the liver and gallbladder to restore equilibrium and optimal performance. Complete guidelines for the liver/gallbladder flush are in Appendix C.

Let's Talk Colon Health

Digestion starts in the mouth. Make sure you chew your food thoroughly. Drink plenty of water throughout the day, but not with your meals. Water with meals will dilute the digestive juices and pH in your stomach. Your goal is to promote absorption of nutrients while rejecting the toxic waste material and by-products. This is one reason for avoiding refined wheat; it coats the digestive track.

The colon is a very sterile environment. It is lined with tiny, finger-like projections called villi, which serve to absorb nutrients. These villi can be destroyed by alcohol, drugs, or chemicals. Coating of the digestive tract, such as can happen by eating too much wheat, inhibits the ability of villi to absorb nutrients adequately.

Why is colon cleansing so important? Because nutrients are absorbed in the colon. Your body, of course, gets nutrients from the food you eat, the water you drink, and the air you breathe. Poor bowel movements, a heavy diet of refined foods, and lack of fiber all negatively impact the colon. A key factor in colon (and overall) health is how fast food moves through the colon. You don't want it to be slow. For the average American, the transient time for food in the colon from consumption to elimination is 96 hours. Ideally, waste elimination should occur within 24 hours. A transient time of 36 hours or more increases the chances of the growth of parasites.

What happens with stagnant colon function? Here are the most significant issues:

- Poisoned brain/nervous system: depression, irritability.

- Poisons to the heart: loss of heart muscle strength, listlessness.

- Poisons to the lungs: foul breath.

- Digestive poisons: bloating.

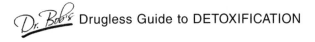

- Blood poisons: sallow, unhealthy skin.

Additional problems may include stiff joints, pain, neuritis, dull eyes, a sluggish brain, and loss of pleasure with life.

You need to create new habits. You want to clear your bowels. You want to get rid of the accumulated waste. That's one of the reasons you might want to get a colonic irrigation.

What you can do:

- Practice better digestion habits by thoroughly chewing your food.

- Eat food your body can use—raw versus fried.

- Eat to live, not live to eat.

- Eat quality versus quantity.

- Enhance bacteria action in the colon. Do not hamper it with chemicals.

- Limit food one day a week. Simply cut back. Limit your food intake one day a week, which will give your colon a rest.

Once you start to cleanse your colon naturally through better food choices, purer water, and more exercise, at first you may notice a variety of body signals, including:

- More bowel movements that are foul smelling.

- Cold or flu-like symptoms.

- Skin breaking out.

- Tiredness.

- Weakness.

- No desire to exercise.

- Depression.

- Nervousness.

These are normal responses to the body throwing off toxins, very much like withdrawal. Do not attempt to stop those signals with drugs.

If you eat a lot of carbohydrates, especially grain products, your colon can become too alkaline. This could result in constipation. The solution? Eat Dr. Bob's ABCs every day. And don't forget cabbage, cauliflower, broccoli, green beans, asparagus; use your imagination.

Just Tell Me What to Do!

In summary, here are the basic detoxification steps you should consider:

- Cut back on the amount of processed food you eat.

- Drink water from a pure source.

- Eat whole foods—raw, steamed, or lightly sautéed with olive oil—whenever possible.

- Bounce on a large ball to stimulate your lymphatic system.

- Chew your food thoroughly.

- Do not drink a lot of fluid with your meals.

- Use the Castor Oil Pack.

- Have your colon irrigated.

- Have your liver/gallbladder flushed.

- Have an herbal cleansing.

- Have your thyroid function tested.

- Avoid alcohol.

- Cut back on coffee and tea; drink decaffeinated preferably Swiss water processed sourced.

- Avoid carbonated sodas.

- Avoid wheat.

- Avoid sugar.

- Avoid dairy products.

Endnotes

1. Hari Sharma, MD and Rama K Mishra G.A.M.S. with James G. Meade, PhD, *The Answer to Cancer: Is Never Giving it a Chance to Start* (New York: Select Books, 2002), 6.

2. Gina Nick, PhD, ND, *Clinical Purification* (Brookfield, WI: Longevity Press, 2001).

HERBS FOR LIFE

Natural healing is like a symphony when all the elements work together in harmony to produce the beautiful result of holistic health. In this symphony, herbs provide a major motif. We need to develop the mindset of taking herbs not just for the sake of symptomatic care but also for creating whole-body wellness.

Let me explain.

The Art of Simpling

Herbology used to be called "simpling." Herbs were known as "simples" because a single herb could be used to treat a wide variety of maladies. The main challenge of herbology for most people today is knowing which herbs to take. It's tough to go to a health store and choose from the list of available herbs without understanding what each one does. You probably should not start taking a lot of herbs on any regular basis until you know which ones are best for your particular conditions, as well as the effect they will have on your body.

The Three Principles of Simpling

1. Use herbs that grow locally. The types of illnesses contracted in a particular area are somewhat dependent on the environmental conditions. For example, conditions in the North favor bronchitis, while conditions in the south are conducive for parasites. Each area may have up to a dozen items that may be used to assist the treatment of ailments.

2. Use mild herbs. Mild herbs can be taken freely and will exert a general positive effect on all the body systems, aiding in the

process of healing many different types of afflictions. Thus almost any herb of mild action that grows in the area may be used.

3. Mild herbs must be used in large doses. Since the herb is very mild, only in a large dose will it have the power to overcome most illnesses.

Use of herbs in their purest form may be called for under certain conditions, particularly with people who are:

- Unwilling to use the large doses of mild herbs.

- Impatient for relief of symptoms.

- Eating a diet derived primarily from foods of other climates, foods eaten out of season, or processed foods.

- Unwilling to devote the time and energy to identify and gather local herbs.

Personally I recommend that you keep on hand a personal "herb box" stocked with such basic herbs as basil, parsley, chives, oregano, fennel, dill, and dandelion root/leaf, preferably grown in organic soil. These are always superior to herbs from an unknown source. I have found from experience when you eat fresh herbs with your salads and meals, your body will respond with vibrant health.

When you eat fresh herbs with salads and meals, your body will respond with vibrant health!

Because of our busy schedules, most of us will find it challenging to do all the necessary homework and legwork to become knowledgeable in the selection and use of herbs, but the result will be well worth the effort. Keep in mind, however, that for any herb to be effective, the various components of our lifestyle, particularly diet and exercise, must be such as to encourage the greatest balance within the body. In other words, the use of herbs will not compensate for a continuing unhealthy diet and lack of exercise.

So often I see people eat with reckless abandon, unwilling to make necessary dietary changes, and yet they want and expect the herbs to bring about a recovery from their ailments. Just as important as the herbs is the act of minimizing or eliminating sugar, wheat, stress, soy, dairy, chemicals, and any other artificial additives such as artificial sweeteners. According to author Michael Tierra L.A., O.M.D, "The main problems that arise in the use of herbs are lack of commitment, lack of consistency, insufficient or extreme dosage, a formula that is not specific enough and last, but perhaps most important, a wrong diet."[1]

Duration of Treatment

For most acute ailments, a good number of people will obtain favorable effects in just three days by using herbs and making appropriate adjustments in the diet and other components of the lifestyle. You may take an herb for up to three weeks; however, if you do not detect changes in three days you may want to change the herb.

As a general rule of thumb, people can expect to require about one month of treatment for every year the disease has been developing.

Like nature, the human body functions cyclically. Our heavenly Father built a seven-day cycle into all His creation. For this reason, herbal treatment works best on a similar cycle. One day out of every seven, do not take any herbs at all. As much as possible, make it the same day each week, in order to preserve the seven-day cycle.

Three Functions of Herbs: Basic Thoughts for Herbal Use

Herbs have three general functions in the body and are compounded according to the state of the individual:

1. Eliminating and detoxifying: using eliminative herbs that act as laxatives, diuretics, diaphoretics, and blood purifiers.

2. Maintaining: using herbs that counteract the physical symptoms, allowing the body to heal itself.

3.   Building: using herbs that tone the organs.

The first stage in herbal treatment generally is to eliminate, removing toxins that are both a physical cause and a result of a disease. However, this step may cause depletion of energy and therefore should not be used for persons who are weak or who are suffering a long-term degenerative condition. In these cases, herbs should be used that will build up the weakened system, such as those recuperating from disease and those with recurring sickness.

For people suffering long-term degenerative diseases or very severe symptoms of an acute disease, the first step is to use herbs that maintain the body through the crisis and stabilize the condition. Once this has been achieved, it is possible to proceed with the appropriate use of elimination and building.

People who have a diet rich in animal products and refined foods have a special need to eliminate toxins and have a characteristic condition for which leaf and flower herbs are most effective. Others who go to the opposite

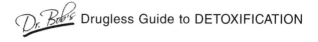

extreme and have a diet rich in raw vegetables and fruits also need to eliminate toxins, as they usually suffer from poor assimilation and are best treated by roots and barks of the herb plants.

Herbs can also be regarded as special foods, and it is often of great benefit to take several herb tonics to aid the major systems of the body. For convenience these are taken in pill or powder form. These tonics bolster the organs of the body and are useful in preventative treatment as well as in the treatment of chronic diseases and congenital weakness.

Someone may, for example, simultaneously take a kidney tonic, a blood purifier, a lower bowel tonic, a glandular-based formula, and an herb tea that is specific for a particular ailment. Such a combination may be taken as a full dose of each tonic separately, or the formulas may be combined to form a single dose that is usually made up of smaller amounts of each component. The former is a full-potency treatment, while the latter is usually satisfactory for long-term treatment and prevention.

Herbal Therapies

There are a number of ways in which the body responds to herbal treatments, and these have traditionally been divided to produce a basis for eight general methods of therapy. These methods are:

1. Stimulation.

2. Tranquilization.

3. Blood purification.

4. Tonification.

5. Control of fluid balance.

6. Sweating.

7. Vomiting.

8. Purging.

Each therapeutic method is suitable for particular kinds of diseases, and it is often appropriate to combine several methods for the most effective treatment.

In applying therapy of any kind, one must regulate the treatment according to the energy of the body. Thus, while the use of certain herbs to eliminate toxins through purging or emesis can be very effective, they are not appropriate for one who is weak or low of energy since these methods will reduce the body energy further. It is important, then, to follow the changing course of the disease each day and to decide which therapy is most appropriate for that condition.

Stimulation

The purpose of this approach is to stimulate the vitality of the body to throw off sickness. Herbal stimulants, when combined with other herbs, will promote their functions of eliminating, maintaining, or building. Effective stimulants include ginger, cayenne, garlic, black pepper, and cloves.

Stimulants increase the metabolism, drive the circulation, break up obstructions, and warm the body. It is particularly useful to apply this therapy in the beginning acute stage of a disease. The body's underlying strength can then be stimulated to throw off the disease.

The herbal stimulants can also restore vitality that has been reduced by chronic illness.

Stimulants can break through blockages and restore balance.

Many ailments are attributed to blockages in the natural flow of blood, lymph, nutrients from digestion and assimilation, water products from food and metabolism or nerve energy. Stimulants are an important means of breaking through these blockages, which are cold, inactive areas of the body. The increase in energy, circulation, and warmth brings back the normal activity. Thus the dynamic balance of all aspects of the physiology may be restored.

Ailments characterized by reduced energy, causing one to feel slow and sluggish, as with colds and the flu, are successfully treated by stimulant therapy, usually in combination with other therapies. In addition, prolonged, low-grade fevers may be treated with warming herbal stimulants such as black pepper and

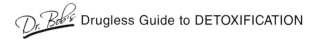

cayenne. I also generally use peppermint leaf any time I have the symptoms of colds or flu coming on.

In this paradoxical situation, *the fever may be neutralized, as the body is aided in its natural production of warmth, thus allowing the fever to subside.* In daily practice I see fevers a lot in people who do not have enough available calcium. Children especially need calcium when they are teething as well as growing. Adults who are under stress need more calcium.

Stimulants are also commonly used to overcome sluggish digestion.

Coffee and tea are also stimulants; however, the main issue with them is that they create an acid environment in the body, which can contribute to other ailments. Do not overuse stimulant beverages—including power drinks and carbonated sodas, whether regular or diet. All of these promote an acidic condition in the body.

Stimulants therapy should not be used when there is an extreme weakness, as often occurs after severe and prolonged disease, since there is not enough basic strength to stimulate to a better action. Stimulants may be added slowly to help other herbs maintain the body through the critical time to rebuild strength. Likewise, stimulants should not be used when the body is eliminating toxins through the skin in the form of eruptive skin diseases, since the use of stimulants will enhance the elimination process and make the disease process appear worse. Minimize stimulants in cases of nervousness and hypertension.

Finally, stimulants, including spicy foods, should be avoided when there is chronic imbalance in the colon. The stimulants will overwork the colon and may lead to problems with the elimination, as well as hemorrhoids. I personally enjoy ginger seeped as a tea, or added to freshly made vegetable juice.

Tranquilization

This therapy is used when there is great unrest, nervousness or irritation interfering

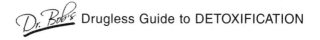

with the process of overcoming the disease condition. In my practice I have seen much unrest with patients who need whole food B vitamins and calcium. Too much stress and too much sugar are common causes. Tranquilizing herbs can be taken over a period of one or two days, and even every hour.

One of three types of tranquiller herbs and foods includes a demulcent that will lubricate joints, bones, and the GI tract. Herbs such as slippery elm bark, marshmallow and comfrey root, and foods like warm organic milk, watery oat, or barley cereals can be used to comfort and quiet a person while the process of healing carries on. Any mucilaginous substance will be effective and may be taken along with warm milk and honey to promote soothing effects.

Nervines are substances that feed the nervous system and balance its energy. These are called nerve tonics. The nervine herbs include skullcap, catnip, wood betony, and valerian.

Antispasmodics calm the nervous tension in the muscles, particularly in the intestines and along the spine. Examples of antispasmodics include lobelia, valerian, kava kava, black cohash, and dong quai.

It is always very important to have adequate calcium in the diet since this strongly affects the function of the nervous system and muscles.

Blood Purification

These are the most significant of all herbs; most herbalists would agree that if you can purify the blood and eliminate acid, the body will function optimally and all diseases will eventually subside.

The blood and lymph system carry a variety of toxic substances. These toxins come from the food we eat, preservatives, and other additives. From my observation, all artificial items need to be processed as foreign invaders. They are not naturally absorbed by the body and often make it so that normal wastes cannot be eliminated properly or with ease.

Traditional Chinese medicine theory suggests that these excess toxins create "heat." Toxin-producing infections are called "hot" diseases. The site of the body most responsible for the purity of blood is the small intestine, which must separate useful nutrients from the totality of substances ingested. Secondary organs affecting blood purity include the liver, kidney, and colon.

There are several ways to purify the blood:

1. Directly neutralize acids with the strong alkalizing effect of some herbs; dandelion and slippery elm.

2. Stimulate the vital organs functions of the body, especially the liver and kidneys, lungs, colon; golden seal and Oregon grape root.

3. Dry excess moisture and remove excess fat where toxins are retained; plantain, mullein, chickweed, and gotu kola.

4. Eliminate excess "heat," especially from the small intestine; rhubarb root.

The best herb for blood and lymph purification is *echinacea*. You can take echinacea daily. I do. It contributes to all the ways blood is purified. Other blood purifiers include burdock root, dandelion, red clover, sarsaparilla, and sassafras.

The best herb for blood and lymph purification is echinacea.

The use of blood purifiers is particularly important for the treatment of infections. Not only does the herb help remove toxins produced by the infection, but it can also remove the excess moisture that provides the medium in which it grows. The infection may be totally eradicated because the herb will stimulate our natural defense mechanism. Echinacea promotes the production of white blood cells, which can then destroy the bacteria and virus.

Tonification

Herbs that build the energy of the organ systems are used as tonics. They are commonly recommended for those who are weak and run down, having low vitality. Tonic therapy is used in the recovery of acute ailments and building energy for those who are dealing with chronic diseases. They are also helpful in maintaining a healthy condition and overcoming minor imbalances.

Tonics are nourishing to the organs; some of the herbs act primarily to provide nutrients; vitamins, minerals, and sugars. The most valuable tonics include sea vegetables, kelp, and Irish moss. Alfalfa, comfrey, and dandelion root/leaf are also useful.

Tonic herbs are used to counteract a deficiency, including weakness or critical shortage in the body. Usually if the body is deficient in one function, there will be deficiencies in all the other functions as well as in vitamins and minerals. Use of strong tonics when one is weak and out of balance is not advisable because they will throw the entire system out of balance. If you are severely out of balance, or if you do not feel good, go slowly. Do not throw strong tonics into your body. Alfalfa and aloe are weak tonics, while dandelion and golden seal are a bit stronger. Any of those may be useful to help rebuild your balance slowly so that your system can tolerate the stronger tonics. I suggest to patients that alfalfa can be taken daily.

Control of Fluid Balance

Body fluids are comprised mostly of water. Through the control of this vital element, we are able to restore and maintain health and wellbeing. The amount of fluids in the body can change very quickly. Our emotions are strongly linked to the balance of fluids in our bodies and thus can also change very quickly. In fact, emotional changes are frequently related to changes in water balance.

Retaining too much water in the body leads to feelings of weakness, paranoia, and depression. Too little water retention, on the other hand, may result in explosive anger and other forceful reactions. Water may be used to quiet the "fire," but too much water will "dampen one's spirits." Excessive water, especially when taken with meals, will disrupt normal digestion by diluting the stomach's acids and enzymes; the internal organs may also become waterlogged. A common example of this is the occasional occurrence of hypoglycemia due to a water-logged pancreas.

Excessive water, especially when taken with meals, will disrupt normal digestion by diluting the stomach's acids and enzymes.

Excessive water can best be eliminated by taking diuretic herbs: horsetail, uva ursi leaves, and juniper berries. The use of these herbs increases the flow of urine, decreases the blood pressure, and helps purify the blood. Diuretics are also useful for weight loss by removing excess water. Vitamin B6 can also be used as a natural diuretic—50 mg three times a day for three months.

If you eat spicy foods, you may be thirsty. Be aware of the amount of fluids you are taking in. Drinking a lot of herbal tea can create too much water in the body. Signs of water overload and stress on the kidneys is bagginess or darkness under the eyes. If you have these body signals, eat less fluid-type fruits and veggies. Parsley supports the kidneys and is helpful in supporting kidney function. It should be seeped as a tea.

Sweating

Sweating is used to treat externally caused diseases such as cold, flu, and fever. Herbs used for sweating are taken as warm teas. The same herbs, taken as cool teas, are useful as diuretics. Sweating occurs to some extent just by drinking the tea but is promoted by providing additional external heat to the body, such as taking a hot bath and then covering up with blankets, after drinking two cups of hot tea.

Vomiting

Emetic herbs induce vomiting and thus quickly empty the stomach of its contents. This may be a necessary treatment if someone is feeling sick from eating too much food or a poor combination of foods.

Some people tend to create excess mucus as a result of certain foods they eat. The first line of treatment is to empty the stomach where the mucus originates. Similarly, emetics can be used to treat colds from overeating.

Ipecac, an herbal syrup found in most drugstores, is an excellent emetic. Lobelia can also be used. Emesis greatly reduces the energy of the body and so should not be used by persons who are already very weak. The emetic treatment may be followed by a mild stimulating treatment, along with soothing demulcent herbs to recover energy.

Purging

Purging by the use of herbal laxatives is valuable in treating ailments associated with the presence of excess secretions, buildup of toxins, or weak elimination. Constipation is considered a serious problem because the retention of wastes in the body can lead to more serious diseases. Purgatives must not be overused, as they deplete the body of energy and thus are only given occasionally to people who are in relatively good health. Proper elimination is very dependent upon the diet and thyroid function.

Herbs work in a number of ways to promote elimination. Some, like cascara bark and rhubarb root, exert a laxative action by stimulating the secretion of bile into the small intestine and increasing the intestinal movement. Others, such as licorice and slippery elm, have a mild action and may be used to treat minor problems in adults or to treat children. Aloe vera combines both these kinds of actions and may be used for more advanced illnesses accompanied by poor elimination.

Bulk laxatives, such as psyllium seed and flax seed, swell up with water and work by greatly increasing the bulk of the intestines.

These herbs are also very nutritive. A combination of these laxatives types, for example, with cascara, licorice, psyllium, flax, and chia, provides a tonic laxative with nutrients, demulcent properties, and stimulation.

Endnotes

1. Michael Tierra, *The Way of Herbs* (New York: Pocket Books, 1998).

2. Daniel B. Mowrey, PhD, *The Scientific Validation of Herbal Medicine* (New Canaan, CT: Keats Publishing).

CASTOR OIL PACK

Before using the Castor Oil Pack, I recommend you discuss it with your natural healthcare provider. You may think that a modality like the Castor Oil Pack is only a cloth with oil on it, but using this low-tech, low-budget procedure, I have seen mononucleosis respond quickly, dysplasia of the cervix return to normal, and digestive distress of long standing normalize. It definitely works, but do not use it without first consulting your health provider.

Castor Oil Packs have been employed for their health benefits since antiquity. Reportedly they were used in ancient India, China, Persia,

Egypt, Africa, Greece, and Rome as well as in North and South America. More modern medical literature indicates their use as a treatment for gastrointestinal problems, lacerations, skin disorders such as psoriasis, as an evacuant, and as a vehicle for introducing medications into the body. Common usage had been for improving elimination capacities, stimulating the liver and gallbladder, healing lesions and adhesions, relief of pain, reduction of inflammation, increasing lymphatic circulation, and drawing acids and poisons out of bodily tissues. Generally speaking, you may wish to employ them to assist your body in its healing efforts in any of these areas.

Necessary Articles

- Castor Oil (100 percent pure, cold-pressed)

- Wool Flannel (cotton flannel should not be used)

- Heating Pad

Procedure

- Fold the wool flannel so that it is three or four layers thick.

- Saturate the wool flannel with castor oil.

- Place the saturated wool flannel in a baking dish and heat slowly in the oven so that the pad becomes hot, but not too hot to place on your skin. Set your oven on low heat and watch your pad carefully and frequently, so it doesn't burn.

- Rub some oil into the skin on your abdomen.

- Lay the warm—not too hot—wool flannel over your abdomen.

- Cover with plastic wrap.

- Cover with a heating pad for one hour. It is important to keep the area as hot as possible. This is why a heating pad is recommended instead of a hot water bottle. A hot water bottle cools too quickly and does not maintain a consistent, hot temperature.

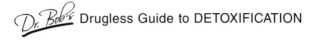

- When finished, remove the flannel and wash your skin.

- Store the flannel in your baking dish covered with plastic wrap or in a zip lock bag. It does not have to be refrigerated. Castor oil is very stable and does not become rancid like other oils.

- If the flannel becomes discolored, other than the normal color of the oil on it, it will probably be due to the drawing of toxins out of the body. When this occurs, wash or discard the flannel.

The flannel can be left on for longer periods if desired. A typical use cycle is three consecutive days per week for as long as is needed—more often if desired.

Castor Oil Pack Benefits[1]

Obviously, conditions known to be related to poor drainage of the lymphatic system will tend to benefit from this type of therapy.

These would include complaints such as:

- Chronic fluid retention accompanied by swollen joints and pain.

- Arthritis.

- Upper respiratory infections involving the sinuses, tonsils, and inner ear.

- Colon problems like Crohn's Disease or colitis.

- Gallbladder disease.

- Boils.

- Liver cirrhosis, hepatitis, enlargement, or congestion.

- Menstrual-related congestion.

- Appendicitis.

- Hyperactivity.

- Constipation, bowel impaction, or adhesions.

- Swollen lymph nodes.

- Bladder and vaginal infections.

I really encourage my patients of both sexes to use the Castor Oil Pack as a regular part of their preventive maintenance program. It is a low-budget, low-tech, highly effective system that promotes liver function. I have had patients with severe mononucleosis respond positively in an amazingly brief time period using the pack. I recommend that you consider using it as a weekly protocol.[2]

Castor Oil

Let's talk about castor oil on its own. It may seem like an "exotic" approach to increase immune system efficiency, but in reality it is a simple modality to improve function without potential negative side effects like the ones that accompany virtually every prescription medication available. I have used castor oil in my practice since the late 1970s and the only side effect I have ever heard of is that the patient's clothes may get oily. This is why I suggest that patients have a "castor oil outfit" consisting of shorts and a T-shirt.

In many ways, castor oil is a unique substance. While most of us are familiar with its uses as a remedy for constipation, folk healers in this country and around the world have used castor oil to treat a wide variety of conditions. Its effectiveness is probably due in part to its peculiar chemical composition. Castor oil is a triglyceride of fatty acids. Almost 90 percent of its fatty acid content consists of ricinoleic acid. Ricinoleic acid is not found in any other substance except castor oil. Such a high concentration of this unusual, unsaturated fatty acid is thought to be responsible for castor oil's remarkable healing abilities.

Ricinoleic acid has been shown to be effective in preventing the growth of numerous species of viruses, bacteria, yeast, and molds.[3]

This would explain the high degree of success in the topical use of the oil for treating such ailments as ringworm, keratoses (noncancerous, wart-like skin growths), skin inflammation, abrasions, fungal-infected finger and toenails, acne, and chronic pruritus (itching). Generally, for these conditions the area involved is simply wrapped in cloth soaked with castor oil each night, or if the area is small enough, a castor oil soaked Band-Aid can be used. (For persistent infections and those finger and toenails that have discolored and hardened, a good 10- to 20-minute soak in Epsom salts prior to applying the castor oil usually speeds up the healing process.)

Castor oil's antimicrobial activity, while very impressive, comprises only a small part of the story concerning this mysterious oil. While castor oil has been thoroughly investigated for its industrial uses, only a minimal amount of research effort has been directed toward its medicinal benefits.

While all of these uses of castor oil are very interesting, the most exciting use deals with ways to increase topical absorption through the use of castor oil packs or poultices.

Much of the current use of castor oil packs in the United States can be attributed to prior natural healing individuals. Time after time they recommend their use based on reports used over the years by many natural healers.

The technique is still practically unknown and shunned by most healthcare professions today. This is probably due to two reasons. First, it's just too simple. It's hard for most people to imagine that something as simple as castor oil packs could have a profound effect on any health problem. Second, in our present health-care system, positive results alone do not constitute the critical factor in determining whether a treatment will be accepted by the medical establishment. Everybody, except probably the patient, now seems to be more concerned about how something is *supposed* to work than whether it actually works at all.

Castor oil packs improve the function of the thymus gland and other areas of the immune system. In my experience, patients using abdominal castor oil packs had significant increases in the production of lymphocytes. Lymphocytes are the disease-fighting cells of our immune system. They are produced and housed mainly in our lymphatic tissues. This includes the thymus gland, the spleen, the lymph nodes, and the lymphatic tissue that lines the small intestine.

Other than knowing it produces the body's white blood cells, most doctors are not very knowledgeable about the lymphatic system. The lymphatic system is an amazingly complex structure. It works hand in hand with both the blood circulatory system and the digestive system. The lymphatic system is the pathway that excess protein molecules can use to return to the circulatory system. Also, along these lymphatic tubules you will find bulb-shaped masses called lymph nodes, which act as filters and produce antibodies when foreign proteins are encountered. Regardless of the health problem, most doctors generally assume the lymphatic system is working accurately, except when someone has cancer.

When castor oil is absorbed through the skin, several extraordinary events take place. The lymphocyte count of the blood increases. This is a result of a positive influence on the thymus gland and/or lymphatic tissue. The flow of lymph increases throughout the body. This speeds up the removal of toxins surrounding the cells and reduces the size of swollen lymph nodes. The end result is a general overall improvement in organ function with a lessening of fatigue and depression.

Your small intestine will become more efficient in the absorption of fatty acids, which are essential for the formation of hormones and other components necessary for growth and repair.

Rubbed or Massaged Directly Into the Skin

Castor oil can be used as massage oil that seems to be especially effective when applied along the spinal column. If the oil is massaged into the body, the direction of the massage should always follow the same path as the underlying lymphatic drainage system, which generally travels from the distal or farther part of the body inward; foot to hip or hand to shoulder.

Conditions Responding to Simple Topical Application

Oftentimes there is no need for castor oil packs; amazing results can be obtained by simply applying directly to the skin. The following is a short list of some of the more common ailments remedied by castor oil:

- Skin keratosis

- Wounds

- Sebacecous cysts

- Muscle strains

- Ringworm

- Bursitis

- Warts

- Itching

- Fungal and bacterial infections

- Abdominal stretch marks; liver or aging spots

- Ligament sprains

Endnotes

1. David Williams, "Castor Oil—Natural Protection from Deadly Viruses" *Alternatives Newsletter; ALTERNATIVES* v 6 n1, July 1995.

2. Clinical-based experience and *Dr. Bob's Drugless Guide to Balancing Female Hormones.*

3. http://www.castoroil.in/reference/glossary /castor_dictionary.html.

LIVER FLUSH

Gall bladder distress can create much pain. With a liver flush you can pass material and residue with ease. I generally suggest patients use the Castor Oil Pack to "soften" the liver up prior to attempting a flush. As with the Castor Oil Pack, consult your doctor before performing the liver flush.[1]

1. Drink one quart of apple juice from the health food store throughout each day for three days. Add 90 drops of *phosfood liquid* and 20 drops of peppermint leaf to each quart of apple juice. The pectin in the apple juice and the *phosfood liquid* helps to soften and flatten thick pasty bile in the gall-

bladder and liver. The *peppermint leaf* will aid digestion. Eat as normal these three days, but for your evening meal on the third day, you may want to eat a light dinner, as you will be drinking the olive oil mixture before bed that evening.

If you cannot tolerate that much fruit juice, or are diabetic, use distilled water instead of apple juice. If you use water, you must increase the amount of *phosfood liquid*. Put 135 drops of *phosfood liquid* and 20 drops of *peppermint leaf* in each quart of water and drink one quart throughout each day for three days.

2. On the third day after the last meal (before bed), mix the following foods together: one cup of high-quality olive oil and one cup of pineapple juice, grapefruit juice, and/or natural spritzer. Add the juice of one whole lemon (organic is best). Stir this mixture together and drink. The pineapple juice or spritzer serves to help get the olive oil down. You will hardly even taste the olive oil. (This program originally included

Epsom salt, but that proved too harsh for most people.)

3. Immediately after drinking the olive oil, go to bed for the night. Put your knees up to your chest. Lie on your right side for half an hour. The oil will go to the gallbladder and liver. These organs will not know what to do with all that oil, so they will overcompensate and throw off accumulated bile residue. It will be best for you to lie on your right side for as long as you can while falling asleep.

4. Take herbal laxatives the next morning. The next day, take an herbal laxative to flush the sluggish bile out of the colon.

Additional Tips

1. Colon Cleanse. We have seen better results when patients have a colon irrigation prior to the flush. This clears the pathway for stone elimination. We also encourage you, after your flush, to have

another colonic. If you have regular yearly colonics, I would recommend the colonic after the flush.

2. All females who pass thick pasty bile and are estrogen dominant (determined by saliva testing) should eat beets either fresh raw grated or baked *for three months prior* to the flush. Beets will help soften the liver/gallbladder unit.

3. Frequency. If you are really sick (such as cancer), consider flushing once a month for a few months. Everyone is different. There are no absolute rules. For prevention, flush at least once a year. Others should do it more frequently.

Protocol Options

One thing you may notice is that the bile material oftentimes will be green and float. You might even want to retrieve your results from the toilet and save it in your freezer. Most of your friends will be amazed that you passed thick pasty green sludge naturally.

Experience with patients completing the flush has taught us some fine tuning for better results. It appears that there is no guarantee that you will pass any material from your body. (The green sludge comes out of your rectum, for those of you who have just read about this procedure for the first time.) We have received reports of individuals passing gobs of green sludge requiring several toilet flushings. Careful attention to the following may improve your chances of sludge elimination:

- Females with a fair complexion with freckles and having one or more children would have better results by adding beet fiber and at least an apple a day to their diet. I would minimize cooked food and eat more whole, fresh, raw fruits and vegetables (see special note below) during this time.

  Females on HRT products, birth control pills, or recent long or short-term medication should follow the protocol mentioned above.

  Supplement with a liver formula that has been developed to support a healthy lipid metabolism with the power of select ayurvedic herbs and glands. Take as a dietary supplement.

Anyone with a history of gallbladder surgery would get a better result by following the protocols listed. I would also suggest taking a liver formula which has bile salts in the ingredients. This will assist in the metabolism of fats that may not have enough bile delivered from the liver.

Special note: Gallbladder bile accumulation is the result of eating a high-acid diet. All foods burn to either acid or alkaline ash after digestion. All meat and dairy products, plus nearly all cooked produce, burn to acid. The body needs to stay slightly alkaline to remain in good health. It makes acid as a by-product of metabolism but makes no alkaline. This must come from the diet. If the diet is primarily animal foods and/or cooked produce, the body must rob the bones of calcium (an alkalinizing mineral) to keep the bloodstream from becoming acidic. But before going to the bones, the body raids the gallbladder. From the bile stored there, it removes the organic sodium (another alkalinizing mineral). What is left behind is cholesterol, which hardens into stones. To protect against gallstone formation, change your diet.[2]

Some indicators suggesting that you may benefit from a liver flush include:

- Blood sugar problems

- Chemical sensitivities

- Cholesterol problems

- Digestion problems

- Dizziness and/or the "shakes"

- Dry tongue and mouth

- Elevated bilirubin and/or liver enzymes

- Elimination problems

- Extreme fatigue

- Eye problems

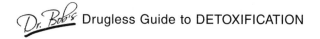

- Female reproductive complaints

- Hair problems

- Headaches

- Mental problems/depression

- Muscle/skeletal problems

- Nail problems

- Pain in the right side of abdomen

- Respiratory problems

- Skin problems

- Susceptibility to infection

- Unexplained weight gain or tendency to gain weight easily

Endnotes

1. Information taken in part from Hulda Regehr Clark's *Cure for All Diseases* (New Dehli, India: Motilal Banarsidass, 2002). Also based on author's clinical-based experience.

2. Taken from Dr. David Frahm's *Health Quarters Monthly,* June 2002. Author of *The Cancer Battle Plan* (New York: Tarcher, 1997).

DETOXIFICATION FOOD SELECTION AND CONSUMPTION

The following are a few basic suggestions to help you stay detoxified:

1. Consume organically grown fruits and vegetables.

2. Obtain fresh produce only in quantities that allow for quick consumption. There is a value to freshness.

3. Always select choice vegetables and fruit.

4. Avoid skinning or peeling vegetables because the skin contains a great part of the nutrients. Try eating squashes, potatoes, and cucumbers with the skin on. Eat

apples, beets, and carrots daily for optimal liver function.

5. Steam or cook vegetables in as small a quantity of water as possible. Do not over cook. Use the juices and the water; you can sip on it as a broth.

6. Eat liberal portions of mixed green salads and raw vegetables twice daily.

7. Eat fresh fruits in season. Focus on pears, plums, and apples only.

8. Substitute frozen fruits when fresh fruits are not available.

9. Eat whole grains. Avoid refined conventional bleached sources.

10. Do what you can to eat whole grain bread. Try spelt, millet, and brown rice.

11. Drink organic milk if you choose to drink milk. I do not personally consume yogurt.

12. Eat organic butter.

13. Confine the number of foods eaten at one meal to a minimum.

14. Eat organic animal tissue and avoid GMO foods.

15. Drink ample amounts of pure water, before or after the meal—minimal fluids *with* the meal. Avoid cold beverages.

16. Use cold-pressed oils, such as olive oil, flax, or sesame seed oils.

17. Drink herb teas instead of soda pop, coffee, or milk. It is easier on the digestive, assimilation, and elimination processes. Use Stevia as a tea sweetener.

18. Eat fruit at least 30 minutes before a meal, never with a meal or soon after a meal. Fruit is digested within 30 minutes, so if it follows food that takes several hours to digest, it will sit in the stomach and ferment. This is another way we cause problems for the colon. I would suggest starting your day with a quartered apple, stewed in the morning with a clove in each quarter. This is an excellent way to stimulate digestion movement and avoid stagnation.

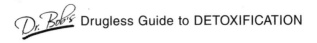

19. Bounce on a large ball or mini-trampoline four or five minutes a day. This will assist in the movement of lymphatic fluids, critical for proper detoxification.

20. Use a shower de-chlorinator and chlorine-free dishwasher detergent to minimize your exposure to chlorine. Also, you will want to limit bromine exposure (white bread, hot-tubs and pools, select beverages). I would locate fluoride-free toothpaste. Make sure you are taking adequate iodine.

Reference: Dr. Cass Igram, *Self Test Nutrition Guide* (Hiawatha, Iowa: Cedar Graphics, 1994), 5223–1548.

PEPPERMINT LEAF

Peppermint leaf, fennel, ginger root, and catnip contain volatile oils and other constituents that absorb intestinal gas, calm upset stomach, inhibit diarrhea as well as constipation, aid digestion, eliminate heartburn, and prevent and remedy childhood colic. These properties are integral to the folk medicine of North and South America, all of Europe and Asia, Africa, Australia, the Pacific Islands—is there anybody left? In tea or capsule, with cream or milk, in small or large quantities, these herbs have served their intended purpose for centuries.

Peppermint is probably the most well-known remedy for stomach problems. Its use can be traced back almost as far as the beginnings of recorded history. It is used for both chronic and acute indigestion, gastritis, and enteritis, acting in two distinct ways to remedy these problems.

1. Peppermint's essential oils enhance digestive activity by stimulating contractile activity in the gallbladder and by encouraging the secretion of bile.

2. Peppermint leaf oils normalize gastrointestinal activity, removing flaccidity and reducing cramps.

Other research has found anti-ulcer, anti-inflammatory, and choleretic principles in this herb.[1] Of no small importance is the ability of peppermint to inhibit and kill many kinds of microorganisms that, among other things, might create severe digestive problems. A few of these bugs need special mention:

•   Influenza A viruses, the cause of much Asian flu.

- Herpes simplex, the source of cold sores.

- Mumps virus.

- *Streptococcus pyogenes*, the cause of sore throat; scarlet fever, rheumatic fever, ottitis media, cystitis, cellulitis, etc.

- *Staphlococcus aureus*, from which we acquire pneumonia, sinusitis, impetigo, endocarditis, etc.

- *Pseudomonas acruginosa*, which produces a great variety of suppurative and other infections.

- *Candida albicans*, the cause of vaginal yeast infection.

Altogether, more than 30 pathogenic microorganisms have yielded to the influence of peppermint.

Endnote

1. Daniel B. Mowrey, PhD, *The Scientific Validation of Herbal Medicine* (New Canaan, CT: Keats Publishing, 1986). Information also from author's clinical experience.

PROBLEM AREAS AND PROGRESS NOTES

_____

_____

_____

_____

_____

_____

_____

_____

_____

_____

_____

_____

_____

_____

_____

_____

_____

_____

_____

_____

_____

_____

_____

_____

_____

Problem Areas and Progress Notes

_____

_____

_____

_____

_____

_____

_____

_____

_____

_____

_____

_____

_____

_____

_____

Other Books by Dr. Robert DeMaria

*Dr. Bob and Debbie's Guide
to Sex and Romance*

*Dr. Bob's Drugless Guide to Balance
Female Hormones*

Dr. Bob's Guide to Stop ADHD in 18 Days

Dr. Bob's Trans Fat Survival Guide

Available From Destiny Image Publishers

Recognized TV Personality • Seminar Speaker • Health Educator

Dr. Bob DeMaria
Your Next Speaker

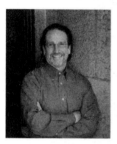

Dr. DeMaria is available to speak at your next Corporate Event, Convention, Community Group or your local church. His energetic speaking style will inspire, educate and motivate your employees or friends to greater levels of health, wealth and personal confidence. Dr. Bob's enthusiasm for life is **contagious**!

Dr. DeMaria is the author of the topselling book "Dr. Bob's Guide to Stop ADHD in 18 Days", as well as "Dr. Bob's Trans Fat Survival Guide", "Dr. Bob's Guide to Optimal Health" and "Dr. Bob's Drugless Guide to Balancing Female Hormones".

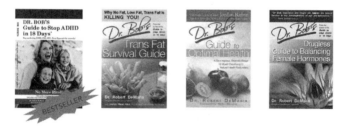

To schedule, contact Debbie DeMaria at 440-323-3841 or fax a request to 440-322-2502 or email your request to druglesscare@aol.com.

Robert F. DeMaria, D.C., N.H.D.

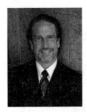

Dr. DeMaria has over 30 years experience as a Natural Health Care Doctor. After graduating with honors from Lorain County Community College, Dr. Bob earned a Bachelor of Science degree in Human Biology, as well as his D.C., from the National University of Health Sciences, **where he graduated cum laude and valedictorian of his class.** He also has a NHD degree from Clayton College. He has his Diplomat Status in Natural Orthopedic Conditions and a Fellowship in Applied Spinal Biomechanical Engineering.

Dr. DeMaria has been recognized as a National and International Natural Healthcare provider by several professional organizations. He is a national and international speaker; author of "Dr. Bob's Guide to Stop ADHD in 18 Days: A Drugless Family Guide to Optimal Health", "Dr. Bob's Trans Fat Survival Guide", "Dr. Bob's Guide to Optimal Health: A God Inspired, Biblically-Based 12 Month Devotional to Natural Health Restoration" and hosts his own TV program. A recognized expert in applied nutrition and human structural biomechanics, he holds post graduate positions and has lectured for the Ohio Supreme Court (CLE credits) and healthcare license credits (CEU).

If you are looking for an exciting presentation that will not only entertain but leave you with viable information to use in your everyday life....

Give us a call – You'll be glad you did!

See Dr. Bob on TV... visit www.DrBob4Health.com.

Ask about our **Employee Wellness Presentations**. Dr. DeMaria can present either a specific topic that you may desire or a series on "Health and Wellness in the Workplace".

To schedule, contact Debbie DeMaria at 440-323-3841 or fax a request to 440-322-2502 or email your request to druglesscare@aol.com.

Additional copies of this book and other book titles from DESTINY IMAGE are available at your local bookstore.

Call toll-free: 1-800-722-6774.

Send a request for a catalog to:

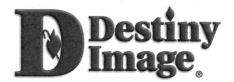

Destiny Image® Publishers, Inc.
P.O. Box 310
Shippensburg, PA 17257-0310

"Speaking to the Purposes of God for This Generation and for the Generations to Come."

For a complete list of our titles, visit us at www.destinyimage.com.